AGENDA

Homage to Geoffrey Hill

AGENDA

CONTENTS

INTRODUCTION		6
Geoffrey Hill:	Some poems first published in *Agenda*	9
HOMAGE		
Geoffrey Hill 1932-2016		16
Robert Richardson:	The Chapter House Reading	21
Stephen Romer:	The Voice of the Heckler	22
David Harsent:	from *Salt*	25
Clive Wilmer:	Geoffrey Hill: Scattered Reminiscences	27
Patricia McCarthy:	Carpenter of Song	32
William Bedford:	Geoffrey Hill: In Memoriam	33
Peter Carpenter:	Geoffrey Hill: The Lost Amazing Crown	34
Peter Carpenter:	Funeral Music	39
Keith Grant:	Geoffrey Hill: a God-given Inspiration	41
Peter Robinson:	Balkan Trilogy	43
Martin Caseley:	Geoffrey Hill: A Reading at Aldeburgh, 2009	45
Omar Sabbagh:	His Solitude	47
Peter Dale:	Two Anecdotes	48
Andrew McNeillie:	Visiting Again	49

POEMS

Rainer Maria Rilke:	Buddha ('Als ob er horchte') Buddha in Glory translated by **W D Jackson**	54
Rainer Maria Rilke:	'You, lost in advance' translated by **Will Stone**	57
Carol Rumens:	Collection Plate Nant y Garth	58
Angela Readman:	The Crows Invite Us to Grieve The Bees Sing Our Night Songs	59
Gill McEvoy:	Growth Rings In Red and White	61
Seán Street:	Mozart's Starling	62
Jeremy Hooker:	Greenfinches The Green Woodpecker Blackthorn and Celandine	64
Peter McDonald:	Weavely Furze Newcastle Island, British Columbia 2015	69
Louis Aragon:	I think of you, Robert (Desnos) translated by **Timothy Adès**	72
Graham Hardie:	The sea of Eden's garden	74
David Pollard:	Rodrigo at the Keyboard A Virginall	75
Jeremy Page:	Leaving	77
Elizabeth Barton:	Now You're Back Swallowtail	78
Dylan Jones:	Acres Cat's Ears	80
David Attwooll:	Otmoor	82
W S Milne:	Torry	84
Angela Kirby:	The Railings Thunder	85

ESSAYS

John Robert Lee: The Sacred in Poetry 88

W S Milne: A Brutal and Primitive Power: 92
The Poetry of Richard Eberhart

Tony Roberts: Al Alvarez at Risk 97

POEMS

William Bedford: The Flitting (i.m. John Clare): 106
Four poems

Vuyelwa Carlin: Scarista Beach, Isle of Harris 110

Sharon Black: West Highland 111

Anne Ryland: The Singing Women of Duddo 112
My daughter no longer needed me
to read her stories

Paul Murray: The Spirit Eel 114

Rosalind Hudis: What the Burglar Took 115

Nick Burbridge: Matriarch 116
Arcadian

John Mole: Across the World 120
The Counterpoint

Jill Townsend: Water Torture 122
Surfacing

David Cooke: Ode to Cobalt 124

Christopher Meredith: In this still air the turning trees 126

Tim Murdoch: Villanelle 127

Gill Learner: Heiligenstadt and After 128
The Genius from Pisa

Peter Dale: Smithereens 130

William Oxley: On a Blackbird Nesting in my Garden 131

Omar Sabbagh: The Bird In The Tree 132

CHOSEN BROADSHEET POETS

Patrick Wright: The Ghost Room   134
                               Nullaby
                               Elisions

Sarah Lindon: I am a group of shadows   138
                               Sunplay
                               Bat
                               Cricket

NOTES FOR BROADSHEET POETS

A few notes from the editor:
The School boy Geoffrey Hill   142

Omar Sabbagh: a close look at   145
Geoffrey Hill's 'Genesis'

Shanta Acharya on *Daodejing* by   149
Laozi – a New Version in English
by Martyn Crucefix

Yves Bonnefoy June 24th, 1923 – July 1st, 2016   154

BIOGRAPHIES   156

Front cover: Portrait of Geoffrey Hill by **Keith Grant**
Artwork in these pages also by Keith Grant.

Courtesy of Keith Grant and the Chris Beetles Gallery, St James's, London

This portrait is the result of the meeting of two great artistic talents. As Artist-in-residence to Keble College, Oxford, and Oxford Professor of Poetry, Keith Grant and Sir Geoffrey Hill engaged in a series of seminars on creativity from 2012, and became friends. Sir Geoffrey then insisted that Keith paint his portrait.

Though best known for his landscape paintings, Keith has produced a number of significant portraits, including those of the Nobel prizewinning chemist, Sir Geoffrey Wilkinson (1988), and Prince Andrew (1994). He has also honoured creative figures either by dedicating works to them or responding to their inspiration in homages.

David Wootton

Introduction by Patricia McCarthy

Words clawed my mind as though they had smelt
Revelation's flesh.

Geoffrey Hill

Geoffrey Hill has long been associated with *Agenda* and highlighted as being the most formidable, challenging, important English poet of our day, or indeed of any day. Upon William Cookson's death in January 2003, he even wrote for William an elegy:

Wild Clematis in Winter

i.m. William Cookson

Old traveller's joy appears like naked thorn blossom
as we speed citywards through blurrish detail –
wild clematis' springing false bloom of seed pods,
the earth lying shotten, the sun shrouded off-white,
wet ferns ripped bare, flat as fishes' backbones,
with the embankment grass frost-hacked and hackled,
wastage, seepage, showing up everywhere,
in this blanched apparition.

(2003)

As William Cookson, founding editor of *Agenda*, commented in his introduction to *Agenda: An Anthology: The first Four Decades 1959-1993* (Carcanet Press, 1994), 'I also put in two short notes on Geoffrey Hill to manifest the beauty of his poetry and its accessibility. They seek to counter the false belief that it is "difficult"'. He quotes Geoffrey Hill: 'Writing poetry is like juggling with conflicting forces in a tiny unit'. A little further on, Peter Dale, writing on Geoffrey Hill, concurs with Pound: 'If poetry reveals to us something of which we are unconscious, it feeds us with its energy'. Rather than expressing the predictable, poems should 'seek to carve out a shape in the unknown'. And this is surely what Geoffrey Hill's poetry does. Alan Massey pays him a great, well-deserved tribute: 'The best language sings from a very small number, and Geoffrey Hill is our most noteworthy *rara avis*.' Similar is Heather Buck's praise. She speaks of his 'passionate voice of warning in our torn and broken world, anger for the selfish indifference toward violence and suffering, as well as affirmation of the beauty of the natural world'. Though written in 1992, she proves how relevant his work is then and now, so that he speaks out of timelessness to all humankind. Regarding the 'difficulty' with which his poetry is too often associated, there is no doubt that his latest works, though highly erudite in their research, became increasingly hermetic, Heather Buck confirms: 'His is the haunted voice of the seer. It is evident that such a voice should attract an avalanche of words, but luckily what he is saying, and the way that he says it, is too important to be eroded by the smoke and stridor of contemporary criticism. There is nothing "difficult", "cold" or "tight-lipped" about his poetry; several re-readings of any page… will yield all the passion and beauty one could desire. Let us pay this great poet, living and writing among us, the tribute of reading his words'.

Christopher Ricks who has written 'such sayings' about Hill's poems down the decades, affirms that they 'matter increasingly; they accrue', and continues: 'Hill is his own man, yet his poems bear witness to T S Eliot's high sense of tradition: The existing monuments form an ideal order among themselves, which is modified by the introduction of the new (the really new) among them. In 1968, *King Log* was the really new. And still is. But then so was all that Geoffrey Hill created on poetry's behalf, on his own dear behalf, and on ours.'

Hill was a very private person and it can be said that, in what he himself called his 'florid, grim music', pitched high, with what Charles Tomlinson called 'his humanising intellect', he sacrifices his real self and causes the death or decreation of selfhood for which he has little regard. Critics will write forever about his intense work, both his uncompromising poetry with its assimilation of history that he makes relevant to any time, his essays, and his complex style with its 'antiphonal ironies, its paradoxes, puns, renovated clichés' (Clive Wilmer). However, will anyone ever be able to fully define the living, profoundly plumbing poems that articulate, as no other has, our human predicament here on earth and our quest, through belief and disbelief, for meaning?

Agenda's business has never been to promote the merely fashionable and ephemeral in poetry; hence the importance of *Agenda*'s promotion of Geoffrey Hill. As William Cookson said: 'Lasting poetry remains timeless and is therefore always contemporary – it does not date, like the ephemera – often the most popular in whatever era… One of the aims of *Agenda* should be to take a stand against the trivia, cleverness, dull predictability – emotion without intellect, fancy without imagination – that pervades much widely praised, and award-winning, current poetry'. *Agenda* remains the same today.

It might seem, then, too audacious a task to compile this special issue in honour of Geoffrey Hill, and we would do best to nod our heads in a reverend silence, as many do. However, it is humbly hoped that the tributes here, whether elegies or pieces of prose, the powerful portrait painting, and the images in black and white – all by Keith Grant – and indeed the poems in general written before Geoffrey's death form a respectful wreath for his fierce and dear shade.

Christopher Ricks called him long ago 'a poet at once urgent and timeless'. Peter Levi summed him up as 'the great cellist of contemporary poets'.

Requiescat in pace.

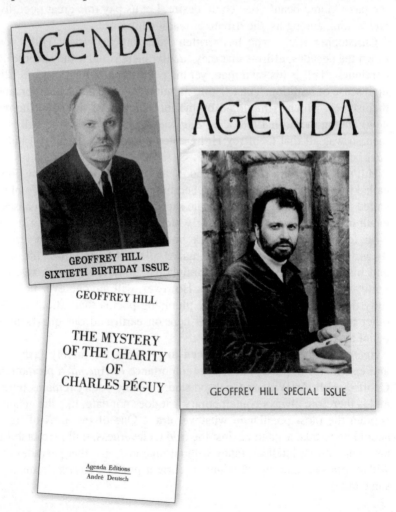

AGENDA

GEOFFREY HILL
SIXTIETH BIRTHDAY ISSUE

GEOFFREY HILL

THE MYSTERY
OF THE CHARITY
OF
CHARLES PÉGUY

Agenda Editions
André Deutsch

AGENDA

GEOFFREY HILL SPECIAL ISSUE

Some poems by Geoffrey Hill
first published in *Agenda*

The Stone Man, 1878

for Charles Causley

Recall, now, the omens of childhood:
The nettle-clump and rank elder-tree;
The stones waiting in the mason's yard:

Half-recognised kingdom of the dead:
A deeper landscape lit by distant
Flashings from their journey. At nightfall

My father scuffed clay into the house.
He set his boots on the bleak iron
Of the hearth; ate, drank, unbuckled, slept.

I leaned to the lamp; the pallid moths
Clipped its glass, made an autumnal sound.
Words clawed my mind as though they had smelt

Revelation's flesh... So, with an ease
That is dreadful, I summon all back.
The sun bellows over its parched swarms.

(1965)

From the *Songbook* of Sebastian Arrurruz

1

Ten years without you. For so it happens.
Days make their steady progress, a routine
That is merciful and attracts nobody.

Already, like a disciplined scholar,
I piece fragments together, past conjecture
Establishing true sequences of pain;

For so it is proper to find value
In a bleak skill, as in the thing restored:
The long-lost words of choice and valediction.

(1966)

From *Lachrimae*

7 Lachrimae Amantis

What is there in my heart that you should sue
so fiercely for its love? What kind of care
brings you as though a stranger to my door
through the long night and in the icy dew

seeking the heart that will not harbour you,
that keeps itself religiously secure?
At this dark solstice filled with frost and fire
your passion's ancient wounds must bleed anew.

So many nights the angel of my house
has fed such urgent comfort through a dream,
whispered 'your lord is coming, he is close'

that I have drowsed half-faithful for a time
bathed in pure tones of promise and remorse:
'tomorrow I shall wake to welcome him.'

(1975)

Terribilis est locus iste

Gauguin and the Pont-Aven School

Briefly they are amazed. The marigold-fields
mell and shudder and the travellers,
in sudden exile burdened with remote
hieratic gestures, journey to no end

beyond the vivid severance of each day,
strangeness at doors, a different solitude
between the mirror and the window, marked
visible absences, colours of the mind,

marginal angels lightning-sketched in red
chalk on the month's accounts or marigolds
in paint runnily embossed, or the renounced
self-portrait with a seraph and a storm.

(1975)

From *An Apology for the Revival of Christian Architecture in England*

7 Loss and Gain

Pitched high above the shallows of the sea
lone bells in gritty belfries do not ring
but coil a far and inward echoing
out of the air that thrums. Enduringly,

fuchsia-hedges fend between cliff and sky;
brown stumps of headstones tamp into the ling
the ruined and the ruinously strong.
Platonic England grasps its tenantry

where wild-eyed poppies raddle tawny farms
and wild swans root in lily-clouded lakes.
Vulnerable to each other the twin forms

of sleep and waking touch the man who wakes
to sudden light, who thinks that this becalms
even the phantoms of untold mistakes.

(1977)

Sobieski's Shield

i

The blackberry, white
field-rose, all others
of that family:

steadfast is the word

and the star-gazing planet out of which
lamentation is spun.

ii

Overnight   as the year
            purple   garish-brown
aster   chrysanthemum
            signally restored
to a sustenance of slant light
as one would venture
                Justice Equity
or Sobieski's Shield even
                    the names
and what they have about them dark to dark.

(1992)

From 'De Jure Belli Ac Pacis'

i.m. Hans-Bernd von Haeften, 1905-1944

iv

In Plötzensee where you were hanged
                              they now hang
tokens of reparation and in good faith
compound with Cicero's maxims, Schiller's chant,
your silenced verities.
                    To the high-minded
base-metal forgers of this common Europe,
community of parody, you stand ec-
centric as a prophet. There is no better
vision that I can summon: you were upheld
on the strong wings of the Psalms before you died.
Evil is not good's absence but gravity's
everlasting bedrock and its fatal chains
inert, violent, the suffrage of our days.

(1994)

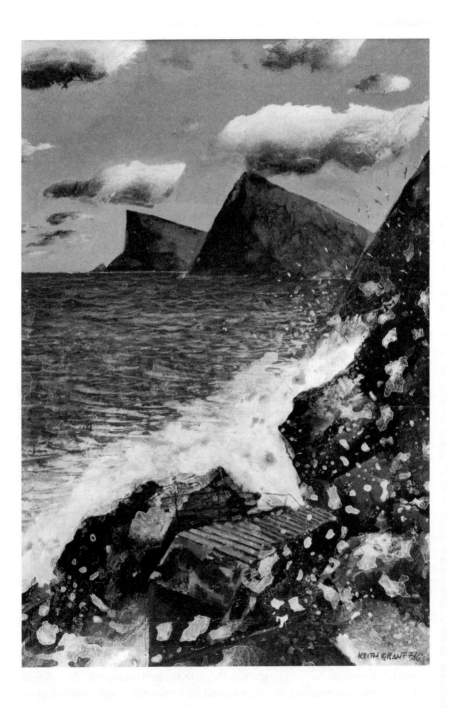

Geoffrey Hill: 1932–2016

It was with great sadness that we heard of Geoffrey Hill's passing on 30 June. His wife, Alice Goodman, posted: 'Please pray for the repose of the soul of my husband, Geoffrey Hill, who died yesterday evening, suddenly, and without pain or dread'. That was good to hear – pain and dread often having featured in Geoffrey's writing and in his life, preoccupations most famously rendered in the lines from 'Funeral Music':

> If it is without
> Consequence when we vaunt and suffer, or
> If it is not, all echoes are the same
> In such eternity. Then tell me, love,
> How that should comfort us – or anyone
> Dragged half-unnerved out of this worldly place,
> Crying to the end, 'I have not finished'.

Or those in *The Mystery of the Charity of Charles Péguy*:

> The blaze of death goes out, the mind leaps
> for its salvation, is at once extinct;
> its last thoughts tetter the furrows, distinct
> in dawn twilight, caught on the barbed loops...

Yes, Geoffrey's mind often ran on last things. Later, in his magnificent verse translation of *Brand*, he would ameliorate the despair by counterpointing the line 'He is the God of Love' to the anguished cry of 'Answer! What do we die to prove?/Answer!' And it would appear that it was in such a state of comfort that Geoffrey passed out of this world.

There was no poet of our time who was more religious in nature, though that nature was often struggling and difficult. In his early years he found composition very hard, publishing a book of verse only once a decade. He became more prolific from his middle years onward as his depression was diagnosed and medically treated. It is not this kind of difficulty that some associate with his work, however, but its seeming intellectual aloofness, especially, it was maintained, in the later works, largely written in the USA. This criticism is otiose, and was finely dismissed by Rowan Williams in his *Guardian* obituary. Geoffrey's 'difficulty', he wrote, 'far from it being a mark of elitism or contempt for the simple and innocent, is a fierce defence precisely against the worst kind of contempt – self-interested or manipulative collusion with what you imagine is the capacity of the public. Just now, when our country has experienced one of its most shameful periods of patronising and dishonest collusiveness, Hill's loss should be felt all the more acutely.' At this point he could have quoted some lines from Hill's 'To the High Court of Parliament':

Where's probity in this –
    the slither-frisk
to lordship of a kind
as rats to a bird-table?

Was Swift ever fiercer? I remember him reading those words in The British Academy one winter afternoon (he was the guest poet at the celebrations for the four hundredth anniversary of John Milton's birth) glaring aggressively across at Pugin and Barry's 'high lamp', as he called it, snarling contempt and writhing his face, spitting the words at the window. Once you heard him read, you knew for certain what poetry was, a force to be reckoned with. And it was equally so on the page, of course.

    I first encountered Geoffrey's poetry as an undergraduate at Newcastle University in the mid-nineteen seventies. Michael Dowd from Coventry, a keen Midlander, introduced me to his work, and after reading *Mercian Hymns* I was certain I wanted to write an MA dissertation on his poetry and prose (apart from being a great poet, Geoffrey, I was convinced, was also our finest living critic). Under the supervision of Dr Desmond Graham and Mr Edwin Morgan I started the thesis in 1977, with helpful assistance from Hill (lecturing at Leeds University at the time) through correspondence with him, and with archival help from his old Oxford friend, the Newcastle University Librarian, Alistair Elliot. I completed the thesis in 1978, and after a request from William Cookson, sent a review of *Tenebrae* to *Agenda* for inclusion in the Geoffrey Hill Special Issue of Spring 1979. William was a keen admirer of Geoffrey's work from the beginning, and had already published some of his finest poems in the magazine, including 'Lachrimae'. He would go on to publish two further special issues on his work (a distinction granted no other poet) and to publish one of Geoffrey's longest and most profound works, *The Mystery of the Charity of Charles Péguy*, as an Agenda Editions' book. Once the book was printed I recall William telling me in his flat in Battersea that he had received a letter of complaint from Geoffrey, berating the printer for a sloping 'I' in his surname, on the spine of the pamphlet. 'I've looked at this closely', he'd written, 'and it is definitely leaning to the left'. Rarely, I thought, had such significance been given to a single character! It reminded me of the famous proof-reader at

Clarendon Press who, it was rumoured, had written a monograph entitled *The Italicised Comma*. He was pulling our legs, of course, getting us to think of the reverberations of that letter ('I', 'aye', 'eye', and so on) in the way he always did with language. Matthew Sperling in his obituary on Hill (he calls him 'an English European', in the magazine *1843*) chooses the phrase 'chequered England' from *The Orchards of Syon* to illustrate this resonance. The phrase reminds us of how England is parcelled out like Larkin's 'postal districts', of our patchwork fields and towns, of the Chancellor's country residence, of John of Gaunt's 'this blessed plot' in *Richard II*, and possibly, I would add, a nodding acquaintance with Silverstone. This is the poet, after all, who could write: 'The poet is hearing words in depth, and is therefore hearing and sounding history and morality in depth'. It was this insight which led him to deride any critic who was tone-deaf to poetry. I still think *Agenda* can boast the single most devastating comment of Geoffrey's in print – his opinion of Humphrey Carpenter's book on Ezra Pound: 'It is not inevitable that a patron will patronize. Mr Carpenter does so, on occasion, with a genial imperceptiveness that can be more damaging than cruel intent. I see little or no evidence that he understands how poetry is made, what its unique difficulties might be, or how one might speak cogently about it'. It reminds one of another fierce Midlander, of Dr Johnson's letter to Lord Chesterfield, declaring the writer's independence from any aristocratic condescension. But Geoffrey would acknowledge human weakness too, quoting Coleridge's words with approval: 'How deep an insight into the failings of the human heart lies at the root of many words'.

William Cookson told me how Geoffrey had called on him unexpectedly one fine summer's morning with a rucksack on his back, asking him if he'd like 'to trudge with him to Chartres?' Cookson had to turn the offer down (he was en route to The Prince Albert pub) but it was clear, retrospectively, that Geoffrey was on his way to do some footslogging research into Péguy's life, for his forthcoming sequence. Like a Method Actor, he had 'to get the feel of the thing'.

Agenda published other fine poems by Geoffrey, including 'De Jure Belli Ac Pacis' in the German Poetry Special Issue, a homage to the German jurist, Hans-Bernd von Haeften, executed for plotting against Hitler. This sonnet sequence stands with 'Funeral Music' as one of Geoffrey's greatest achievements. Cookson also commissioned some of Geoffrey's finest essays, including 'Our Word is Our Bond', 'perhaps the most searching enquiry into the responsibilities and affordances of writing by any post-war poet', as Matthew Sperling has termed it. Latterly Geoffrey disgraced himself magniloquently as a Knight of the Realm and as Oxford Professor of Poetry (one of the oldest ever appointed).

In the minds of the editors of *Agenda* Geoffrey was simply the finest English poet since Auden, and peerless over the last forty years or so. He was a magnificent poet, unrivalled in his passion for the craft and study of poetry, and his essays I am certain will last as long as his verse. I would rush out to buy a book of his poems or prose as they appeared before any other author's, and it was with a sense of sadness for once that I learned his last book (his verse-translations of Ibsen's *Brand* and *Peer Gynt*, published by Penguin) appeared on the day of his death, a day it seems he had spent shopping for books as usual in Heffers, Cambridge. *Brand* is a reprint with minimal corrections, but *Peer Gynt* is a fresh and new work, a revelation. I think it contains some of his best poetry of recent years. In his last interview Geoffrey says that *Peer Gynt* (like *Brand*) is a theological drama, a genre rare in English literature, with the exception, he says, of Milton's *Samson Agonistes* – although one can argue that Eliot's plays fall into this category. He told Kenneth Haynes that he went to Robert Garioch's Lallans translation of George Buchanan's mid-sixteenth century drama, *Jephtha*, to find a model he could admire at home. The anecdote serves to emphasise the range and depth of Geoffrey's reading and scholarship. His *Peer Gynt* is better than any film (Haynes likens it to a film) for it evinces life in the words themselves, conveying the joy, the high jinks and hubbub of humanity. The 'heft' (it was one of Geoffrey's favourite words) of the translation is that 'To lose all hope of at last returning to God' is a terrible thing, something 'the licensed demons' of our times, the monsters and the trolls (and there are plenty of them in Geoffrey's work) do not understand. They are cast off from the 'grace more enduring even than mortal corruption':

> Lucerna,
> the soul-flame, as it has stood through such ages,
> ebbing, and again, lambent, replenished,
> in its stoup of clay.

They are neglected, abandoned, dancing 'at the grid of extortion', and Hill's translation makes Ibsen current for our day.

The characters Brand and Peer Gynt, with their poetic intensity, pitch themselves against 'a canting, provincial, sanctimonious, murderously self-righteous society' (these are Hill's own words) and their vision, in a way, is close to Geoffrey's own. They seek out God in the most desolate places, as Geoffrey himself had done:

> Below, the river scrambled like a goat
> Dislodging stones. The mountain stamped its foot,

19

Shaking, as from a trance. And I was shut
With wads of sound into a sudden quiet...

Pent up into a region of pure force,
Made subject to the pressure of the stars;
I saw the angels lifted like pale straws;
I could not stand before those winnowing eyes

And fell, until I found the world again.
Now I lack grace to tell what I have seen;
For though the head frames words the tongue has none.
And who will prove the surgeon to this stone?
(from 'God's Little Mountain')

Only a few months ago Geoffrey wrote an essay-review on the life and poetry of Charles Williams for the *Times Literary Supplement*, showing no signs of diminishing powers. He was as alert as ever to the end.

As for Geoffrey's craft, Seamus Heaney had summed it up precisely: 'Hill addresses the language... like a mason addressing a block'; 'words in his poetry fall slowly and singly, like molten solder'. They are fine words from a fellow master.

Geoffrey was proud of his working class origins in Bromsgrove, and said that he had often felt intimidated at Oxford, but when he was viva'd at Keble College for his English degree, he was awarded a First by, amongst others, J R R Tolkien. Tolkien said, 'I like the cut of that young man's jib'. The cut of Hills' jib is evident in some of the finest poems to appear in English since the Second World War.

Let us finish with a memory of Geoffrey's, from the village of Fairfield, witnessing the bombing of Coventry on the night of November 14, 1940:

Coventry ablaze... that armoured
city suddenly went down, guns
firing, beneath the horizon; huge silent whumphs
of flame-shadow bronzing the nocturnal
cloud-base of her now legendary dust...

So it is poetry is made, and remembered.

Geoffrey's poetry will remain when much else will have turned to dust. A great soul has gone out of the world, a friend *Agenda* will miss. English literature has lost a master.

W S Milne

Robert Richardson

The Chapter House Reading

for Geoffrey Hill (at Lincoln Cathedral)

i

Words strict as these blocks of stone
serving their purpose to fit

and so create a structure
where beauty is also shown;

listening was itself a trance
of meaning chipped into sound,

a transfer of the moments
poems were made to enhance.

ii

The Reading came to an end,
words were no longer distinct

but part of a crowd's chatter
that poured out its muddled blend;

you seemed to be a sealed will
defined well against the stone

and contained within a coat
resisted silence's chill.

Stephen Romer

The Voice of the Heckler

The Editor of *Agenda* kindly asks for a piece on Geoffrey Hill, which I must write to a very tight deadline, which exercises the mind. I shall perforce be brief.

What adds to the constraint is my consciousness of the 'voice of the heckler' – that rude, interrupting, querulous voice that became so much an essential part of the armoury of the late poetry. Armoury – in his lecture on Poetry and War in Wolfson College, Oxford, in 2010 shortly before his election as Professor of Poetry, Hill spoke about the latest tank, used apparently by the Israeli Army. (I have this on the word of the historian Patrick Wright – whose book Hill reviewed). This tank is such an efficient and bristling fighting machine that it can, by means of chemical reaction, somehow turn enemy fire back on the enemy. Such should be the modern poem, Hill was saying, a fighting machine, able to wrong-foot and short-circuit any critical tirade that might be made against it. In that magnificent, similarly bristling lecture, I recall he picked out some famous lines of Wilfred Owen's and confessed to his sorrow at having to describe them as very weak indeed. Nothing ever did sit easy with Geoffrey Hill, and never for long.

So this business of an informal piece on him, now that he has died, is particularly fraught. One obituarist picked out 'September Song' from *King Log* as an exemplary 'Hill poem' in which ambiguity is cultivated over double-entendre and line ending. But as recently as April this year, when he gave what turned out to be his last reading at Emmanuel College, Cambridge – truth be told it was more of a theatrical turn, comic and excoriating, and self-excoriating by turns – he picked out that very poem to say how much he *regretted* that it had become so popular. And *why* has it become so popular? Because it is 'good humanitarian *copy*'. Once at a panel discussion with him, at the École Normale Supérieure in Paris, I made some idle comment about how I was grateful for having had the chance to re-read the poet's work – and GH spluttered 'how *dreadful* for you!' And he was explosive at those at the same meeting who wanted to harp on about him as a great 'poet of landscape'. This clearly was not enough, it was idle, it would not do.

Even at his funeral, no one was free from the voice of the heckler, in this case surely his own. At that service, where nothing was wanting in decorum and music, and the language was the sweetest Latin, and the English of the King James Bible and the Prayer Book, there was a reading from *Corinthians* 15... and some lines from *Speech ! Speech !* swam unerringly into my mind – 'When all else fails, CORINTHIANS will be read/ by a man in too-tight shoes.' We have learned, in late Hill in particular, there shall be no 'plateau of reassurance', indeed no resting place, the default position perpetually questing and self-questioning – a lot of finger-pointing, but primarily at himself – 'What is he saying ;/ why is he still so angry ? He says, I cannot/ forgive myself.'

But this is not how I first read Geoffrey Hill, or indeed wanted to read him. In my case (everyone will have a different *introit*) it was 1978, and the publication of *Tenebrae*. Ironically perhaps, I was in the United States at the time, and suffering in the 'dry, secondary air' of a university, and I received his words, especially the sonnets of 'An Apology for the Revival of Christian Architecture in England' like the healing waters.

> On blustery lilac-bush and terrace-urn
> bedaubed with bloom Linnaean pentecosts
> put their pronged light; the chilly fountains burn.

I was in Virginia when I read those words, among the flowering dogwood, and the scarlet cardinals – nothing could be more American, but I was transported back to the houses and churchyards of England. And no one, surely, has captured so much of British India, or ideas about British India, seen through a particular lyrical prism as in the three sonnets that make up 'A Short History of British India', a title that revels in its own hubris.

Geoffrey Hill 'banged on' a great deal about 'fallenness' – the fallenness of language, and the fallenness of man. It is one of his richest veins; he was one of those (like the dejected Coleridge?) who believed in original sin firmly, but in concomitant redemption only fitfully. He decided in *The Triumph of Love* that the poem might be 'a sad and angry consolation' and in lines like this from the 'Tenebrae' sequence

> Staggering images of grief-in-dream
> Succubae to my natural grief of heart
> Cling to me then...

I have found more consolation than in anything more conventionally 'consolatory'. Once I wrote a fan-letter to Hill, a young man's letter flush with enthusiasm that would now make me wince; in any case I dared to compare him to George Herbert and Gerard Manley Hopkins. Entirely characteristic of Hill that he should write back, a densely-written post card, thanking me for the words, but lamenting that – hidden within a Latin quotation from Ovid – 'the healer could not heal himself'. Now he is gone, I am aghast at how his language, great swathes of it, has come to inhabit me, and has enlivened me, and focused my own apprehensions, for so many years. But I hear the voice of the heckler again: how *dreadful* for you!

David Harsent

from *Salt*

i.m. Geoffrey Hill

How fine they are, the things of grossest hurt –
                    (The Daybooks VI: Al Tempo De' Tremuoti)

They found they could let slip their other selves, pale mavericks
who would take to the streets dazzled by liberty, would talk
to anyone, cross at blind corners, bed down in daylight.

*

Her spittle was wine and salt. Later, he took salt
from the tip of her breast with the tip of his tongue.
They could eat whenever they chose, they could go
from room to room without having to say why, or sit
in total darkness close enough to touch but never touching.
They thought they might cut each other's hair to get
the sudden lightness in that, the flow, the naked neck.

First, that grand percussion as the pick-up
swerved and hit; then the creature down, legs
still going at a flat-out run, its tripes starting to spill.
Sunlight on blood and diesel; trees turning in the wind;
the road empty save for this. Finally, he slept.

*

There in a salt-mist, in fever-dreams, his image
caught between the glass and the mirror-back,
powerless, motionless, sightless, breathless, enraged...
The mirror trembles. His eyeballs smudge the skim.

*

A blind house: no door to the world outside,
every window sealed, a web of hallways, rooms
littered with absences. Heartless geometry.
People stand in the street and call your name.

Clive Wilmer

Geoffrey Hill: Scattered Reminiscences

On 28 April this year, in a lecture theatre in Emmanuel College Cambridge, Geoffrey Hill read and talked to a packed audience. It must have been his last reading. During questions, a woman raised her hand to tell him that he was talking too much and reading too little. The speaker turned out to be Hill's wife, Alice Goodman. He was immediately penitent – to some degree mock penitent, perhaps, but none the less conscious that his wife was right. He *had* talked too much. The talk had mostly been good, but the readings were electric. Hill was blessed with a resonant voice, deep musical feeling and a flawless ear for the rhythms of English verse. His poetry lived contentedly – had its full vivid life – within the accepted constraints of those rhythms, but one only had to hear half a line to know whose poems they were. On the occasion in question, for instance, he read 'Merlin' from his first book, *For the Unfallen* (1958):

> I will consider the outnumbering dead:
> For they are the husks of what was rich seed.
> Now, should they come together to be fed,
> They would outstrip the locusts' covering tide.
>
> Arthur, Elaine, Mordred; they are all gone
> Among the raftered galleries of bone.
> By the long barrows of Logres they are made one,
> And over their city stands the pinnacled corn.

I couldn't hear him read his early poems, those I have known since I was seventeen, without coming out in goose pimples. It was and is something to do with the slightly syncopated rhythm – line 7 is a good example – and something to do with the assembly of chromatic rhymes, four to each stanza, only one full rhyme in the whole poem. Then there is the surprisingly formal mode of address: 'I will consider', not 'it seems to me' or 'just think about this'. In his talk Hill picked on the word 'pinnacled' as the one that made the poem and gave it its sense. He was surely right about this. The use of an architectural term – especially one from medieval architecture – preserves the sense of society in the poem, though the city has given way to fields of corn.

There is something about the blend of agriculture, chivalry and Gothic architecture in this poem that reminds me of John Ruskin. For most of my life, Ruskin has been my hero, but I only recently realised that Hill was a fellow enthusiast. This may be something to do with the times we live in – the political and social circumstances that provoked Hill's poems 'To the High Court of Parliament', for instance. It is not widely realised that he wrote the best part of a book about Ruskin's doctrine of intrinsic value, 'Inventions of Value', one of the discrete sections of his *Collected Critical Writings*. In an interview he gave to *The Oxford Student* in 2011, he said: 'I would describe myself as a sort of Ruskinian Tory. It is only Ruskinian Tories these days who would sound like old-fashioned Marxists. I read and re-read Ruskin, particularly *Fors Clavigera*, and I am in profound agreement with William Morris's [lecture] "Art under Plutocracy"'.

The latter is the incendiary attack on capitalism which Morris delivered in Oxford in 1883. On that occasion, many respectable dons stormed out of the room when Morris invited them to convert to Socialism. Order was only restored when Professor Ruskin rose from the floor, defended Morris and identified with his analysis. In late years, Hill would borrow a phrase from Morris's lecture to characterise our modern polity: 'anarchical Plutocracy' he would call it. It is one of the phrases that Ruskin would have found quite easy to endorse.

In the early 1980s – I forget the exact date – I was lucky enough to be able to introduce Hill to one of the modern poets he most admired. This was the American poet Edgar Bowers (1924-2000), whom I regard as one of the finest poets of the last half century. I was enormously pleased to discover that Hill shared my view of Bowers, though his admiration was especially focused on two or three poems from Bowers's first book *The Form of Loss*. Hill was then lecturing in Cambridge and I took Bowers to meet him in his rooms at Emmanuel. I wish to goodness I had kept some record of that conversation. One thing I especially remember. Not long after the two men fell to talking, Hill expressed admiration for Bowers's 'Two poems on the Catholic Bavarians' and recited two or three stanzas from memory.

Thus in the summer on the Alpine heights
A deity of senseless wrath and scorn
Is feasted through the equinoctial nights
As though a savage Christ were then reborn.

Up from the floors of churches in December
The passion rises to a turbulence
Of darkness such as threatens to dismember
The mind submerged in bestial innocence.

And Druid shades with old dementia fraught
Possess the souls they had accounted loss
And join their voices, raging and distraught,
About the curious symbol of the cross.

Hill was word-perfect when he recited this, and the resonance of his voice was exactly appropriate. That same evening, we were treated to a similar recitation from one of the weightier poems of Charles Wesley.

I remember him saying at this time that he found all religious belief fascinating and relished the detail of particular practices and understandings. That was surely part of the appeal of Bowers's poem. Bowers was brought up as a Presbyterian and, though an agnostic, retained a religious temperament. Called up for service in the US army at the end of the Second World War, he had been assigned, aged twenty-one, to the denazification programme based at Hitler's Berchtesgaden. Coming from the deep south and the Bible-belt, he wrote with extraordinary freshness about the Catholic Bavarians. This, I think, is what appealed to Hill.

If I had to name my favourite poem of Hill's, I would probably choose the sixth section of 'Funeral Music':

My little son, when you could command marvels
Without mercy, outstare the wearisome
Dragon of sleep, I rejoiced above all –
A stranger well-received in your kingdom.
On those pristine fields I saw humankind
As it was named by the Father; fabulous
Beasts rearing in stillness to be blessed.
The world's real cries reached there, turbulence
From remote storms, rumour of solitudes,
A composed mystery. And so it ends.
Some parch for what they were; others are made
Blind to all but one vision, their necessity
To be reconciled. I believe in my
Abandonment, since it is what I have.

I believe Hill once said that this sonnet from a poem overtly about the Wars of the Roses was modelled on those poems written on the eve of their execution by condemned noblemen: Chidiock Tichbourne's 'My prime of youth is but a frost of cares', for instance, or Sir Walter Raleigh's 'To his Son'. Here is the latter:

Three things there be that prosper up apace
And flourish while they grow asunder far;
But on a day, they meet all in a place,
And when they meet they one another mar.
And they be these: the Wood, the Weed, the Wag:
The Wood is that which makes the gallows tree;
The Weed is that which strings the hangman's bag;
The Wag, my pretty knave, betokens thee.
Now mark, dear boy – while these assemble not,
Green springs the tree, hemp grows, the wag is wild;
But when they meet, it makes the timber rot,
It frets the halter, and it chokes the child.
Then bless thee, and beware, and let us pray
We part one with thee at this meeting-day.

Raleigh is admonishing a young rascal who happens to be his son. The warning is grim – 'It frets the halter, and it chokes the child' – but it is touched throughout with tenderness. Hill's poem is extremely tender too, though in it the power-relation is more or less reversed. In Hill's poem it is the child who has the power: the power a child has over a loving parent, but also the power of the imagination – 'when you could *command* marvels' and so on. The speaker is briefly admitted to the boy's imaginative world. It reminds me of visiting the bedroom of one's son, perhaps to read a story to him. But the poem reminds *us* that that is a relationship with an inescapable end. It is first disrupted by the sound of other adults – downstairs, perhaps in the street – which comes to the speaker as 'the world's real cries', and then, in the end, he finds himself exiled from paradise. He is 'abandoned', rediscovering himself in 'the desolation of reality' – to borrow a phrase of Yeats's.

I think it must have been while discussing this poem and my attraction to it, that Hill mentioned his love of children's literature. The end of his first marriage had meant separation from his children and he found that one way of maintaining the relationship with his daughter was to send her books and talk and write to her about them. He used to argue that the standard of writing for children in our country was much higher on average than that of literature for adults. Jane Gardam was a great favourite, for instance, but he was also strongly attached to the books he remembered from childhood. I shared one of his passions. It was for the stories of Alison Uttley, the creator of *Little Grey Rabbit*, which I too had known as a boy and more recently read to my daughter. Uttley, he pointed out, had got into his poems. Fellow admirers of her books will remember the story of *Moldy Warp the Mole*, the protagonist of which is a kind of archaeologist who discovers a Roman coin. He turns up in the fourth section of *Mercian Hymns*:

I was invested in mother-earth, the crypt of roots
and endings. Child's-play. I abode there, bided my
time: where the mole

shouldered the clogged wheel, his gold solidus; where
dry-dust badgers thronged the Roman flues, the
long-unlooked-for mansions of our tribe.

As everyone who knew him seems to agree, Geoffrey Hill could be hilariously funny in conversation. I must admit that, on the whole, I like the early poetry better than the late, but if it has a fault of any kind, that fault is surely that its tone is almost invariably solemn. In the later work, with its hecklers and dissenters fully incorporated, Hill is often very funny. He is never quite as funny, though, as he was in conversation.

Five or six years ago I ran into him at a Cambridge garden party. I hadn't seen him for a while and was surprised to discover that he had changed his image. He was dressed very flamboyantly with dandyish precision and he had grown his beard to its full length. It was as blanched and luxuriant as the beard of Father Christmas. I was reminded of Edward Lear:

There was an Old Man with a beard,
Who said, "It is just as I feared! —
Two Owls and a Hen, four Larks and a Wren,
Have all built their nests in my beard.

I mocked him very gently and commented, too, on a splendid new hat that he was wearing. It was strikingly a hat from a different era: black with a stiff, wide brim and a dent made just off-centre in the crown. 'This hat,' he responded, 'represents the swiftest transaction I've ever been party to. I went into a shop in Jermyn Street – a shop famous for its hats – and the assistant asked if he could help. 'Yes,' I said. 'I want to look like a middle-European composer, circa 1928.' 'I have exactly the thing for you, sir!' the assistant replied, and he brought me this hat, which I purchased on the spot.'

I believe there is quite a lot of writing by Hill that has not yet seen the light. I wonder if that anecdote will surface from it.

Patricia McCarthy

Carpenter of Song

i.m. Geoffrey Hill

We met in a palace.
The high heels of the diminutive Queen

tapped the carpet on which your feet,
as if in hobnailed boots, placed their stamp.

On a bare wooden bench you sat,
isolated, shaggy eyebrows grafted together,

still and solid as Rodin's Thinker.
I perched beside you, your profile silhouetted

already in my mind's mirrors. Your measured bass,
worded, cast you as a workman in a back yard,

planing metric lengths for your carpentry
of dovetailed lines, unphased by fairytales

too often reversed. No ermine
upon your shoulders. Yet the blued blood

of Celtic Druids coursed calligraphies through
the veins of your hand I shook; your lineage

dubbed you a Master Bard, silence-shaver.
Such might to carry forever after

whole kingdoms on your back...
Now the sky cracks open

between turreted clouds to welcome you:
death-dealer, angel-flyer, self-struggler,

old as Taliesin, young as an unborn.
While your syntax, in every language at once,

gnarls the trees, the gale-force of your going
knocks us, your acolytes, onto our knees.

William Bedford

Geoffrey Hill

In Memoriam

When Geoffrey Hill died, it was as if somebody I knew had died, and yet I never met him. I felt the same when Ted Hughes and Seamus Heaney died. It's ridiculous in a way, but then I realised that in fact I have been reading Hughes, Heaney and Hill since I was a boy, and in some weird sense I almost know them, or feel that I know them, better than the people I actually do know. It may be that all I know through reading is what Proust calls the poet's 'better self', but that is hardly a bad way to get to know somebody. With Hughes and Heaney, I felt a sense of personal loss. With Geoffrey Hill, the loss is less emotional, more foundational. For decades I have found myself wondering 'What is he saying: / why is he still so angry?' and finding in his poetry and prose, his 'fascination with what's difficult', the tough-minded consolation of the true seer. Finding in 'Funeral Music,' the only answer to the magnificent *laus et vituperatio* of *The Triumph of Love*, the poet 'Crying to the end "I have not finished."' He is not finished, because his work is what we have become.

Peter Carpenter

Geoffrey Hill: The Lost Amazing Crown

A good deal of my life has been shaped by the reading, and consequent study, of Geoffrey Hill's poetry; that reading started around 1973 when I was handed a copy of *King Log* by my English teacher, Kenneth Curtis, (KHMC), to whom the collection was dedicated.[1] My life has been considerably enhanced by this experience, thus Geoffrey Hill's death and the end to any furtherance of his poetic output will inevitably diminish it. His importance to my life and times has gone hand in glove with his poetry's challenges and rewards. I love re-reading Hill's poetry, especially that work I know the best, from *For the Unfallen* (1959) to *Without Title* (2006); and hearing it too, principally via the wonderful Clutag recording I own. I admit too that I count those earlier poems as his greatest achievements. His finest poems have that quality of great art: they are 'shape-shifters' in the mind and heart, perpetually revealing new threads, patterns and puzzles, never exhausted or reducible, enduring as acts of 'sad and angry consolation'.

Passion attracts information, and Hill's work has led me into long-standing friendships with poets and scholars who have recognised Hill's genius. Many readers have been put off his poems by what they perceive as 'difficulty', principally the prickly textures from a latterday modernist that eschew a confessional mode or encourage 'accessible' reading. Then there is the dazzling erudition. The reverse has been true for me. In many poems, essays and lectures Hill put the counter argument with force and sense: why should poetry not be difficult, along with music, sculpture, the visual arts? 'All a poet can do today is warn' were Wilfred Owen's words: many of Hill's poems seem to me urgent reminders or warnings (from history), that go unheeded in our age of sound-bite politics, Brexit and Trumpery. Most are implicit, although some, as in the third part of 'Reading Crowds and Power', are more explicit:

> But hear this: that which is difficult
> preserves democracy; you pay respect
> to the intelligence of the citizen.
> Basics are not condescension. Some
> tyrants make great patrons. Let us observe
> this and pass on. Certain directives

parody at your own risk. Tread lightly
with personal dignity and public image.
Safeguard the image of the common man.[2]

In 2009, Peter Sansom asked me to choose the poetry collection most important to me; *King Log* was an easy choice for its significance beyond itself, emotionally and historically. What I tried to do was to go back to what that first reading experience was like, an attempt I realise itself prone to myth and error. But here is part of this account, intended to show the shock of the 'new':

Everything about the writing puzzled me, but somehow it stuck. The poems were like internal wrangles, contests, debates taking place in miniature, or arguments fused into a language that was by turns spare and stark and then richly textured, sensuous, bloody. Bread and water then venison stew, eel pie. Words and lines with trap-doors. Cryptic clues, dark, bizarre puns. Entire poems and sequences standing seemingly to attention. Who goes there? A twitchy quality: the watch at the start of *Hamlet*. Intimations of some terrible knowledge beyond the comprehension of any reader.

It is hard to cleanse the poems of subsequent critical estimations (there were no 'reader's guides out there then, no York Notes, no Google; no acclaim from apologists). Here are a few of the opening gambits:

'The Word has been abroad, is back, with a tanned look'
('Annunciations')

'Anguish bloated by the replete scream'
('Three Baroque Meditations')

'Processionals in the exemplary cave,
Benediction of shadows. Pomfret. London.'
('Funeral Music')

'So with sweet oaths converting the salt earth
To yield, our fathers verged on Paradise.'
('Locust Songs')

Challenges. Have at thee. The range in tones, the sense of real voices emerging from some drama, the shifts in diction from formal, liturgical cadence to newly-aged colloquialisms: all these qualities simultaneously baffled and intrigued. Poems like controlled explosions. The subject matter was as hard to pin down as the voices, but a sense of grief and grieving, the weighing up of moral responsibilities in the face of violence, violation, horror: these seemed to be central. And history. The Holocaust, the Wars of the Roses (slaughter at the Battle of Towton), the American Civil War, as well as meditations on age and childhood that came from closer to home. Nothing confessional, nothing directly about the poet's emotion, but obliquely a choking or clenching of strong feelings in the face of injustices. Looking back at it I think that this overarching seriousness, the sombre moves in and from other worlds, was very attractive to a teenager weighing up big questions, directionless beyond some sense that there was more to life than suburban Surrey.[3]

My study of Hill's work developed at Cambridge in 1978 when I mentioned to Eric Griffiths that I liked Hill's poetry; *Tenebrae* was published that year, a thrilling event for me and, essentially encouraged by Eric's patient dedication, I took it upon myself to 'read around' all the poems, then all the essays, which I soon discovered to be the matter of a lifetime, (still) shaming my ignorance. The resulting Part Two dissertation ('Brilliance Made Bearable', ha!) was the product of a pre–digital age and a week or so in May 1979 with the cultural guru Kevin Jackson, as he helped me on the Silver Reed, count as one of the more joyous times in my life. Thereafter I met Hill after one of the Clark Lectures in 1985; I bumped into Ken Curtis at the lecture and we walked over together from the Sidgwick Site to Eric Griffiths' rooms in Trinity. I remember that walk with fondness but with no clarity; this was the last time I was to see Ken alive.

In 1988 I moved back to Cambridge and was again in contact with kindred spirits such as Peter Robinson, as well as gaining Clive Wilmer as a neighbour and friend. One of the abiding points of contact was a shared love of Hill's poetry; Hill and Thom Gunn we felt were always seemingly ignored or underplayed in the public eye and the world of letters next to Hughes and Heaney. A simple thing to remark upon here is this: that examination boards have veered away from Hill's poetry and thus diminished his potential readership, depriving a pre-university audience of the chance to be fascinated or perplexed. I have counted it as one of a pleasurable duty in my career to teach some poems by Hill to my students in secondary education; almost unfailingly they rise to the challenge. I have attended many readings by Hill and was lucky enough to catch his last ever public reading at Emmanuel in April. I sat next to Clive Wilmer and Kevin Jackson; behind me was a young student, from Sidney Sussex, and poet, Conor McKee, destined to gain the highest first in his year, who had kept in touch with Hill since days in classes at Tonbridge, and who had chosen the 'Funeral Music' sequence as a text for his Tragedy paper. The news of Hill's death made the circumstances of the reading all the more poignant; the reading itself becoming a matter of awed silence when Hill read and introduced poems such as 'Merlin' and 'Requiem for the Plantagenet Kings'.

I am sure that his poetic achievements will stand the test of time; the poems follow the much-admired and oft-cited dictum from Milton: they are 'simple, sensuous and passionate', their mysteries and powers demand much from the reader, they resist the tyrannies of simplification that lead to political, artistic and philosophical disaster. This makes the whole business sound terribly po-faced: Hill is very funny indeed: he has an ear for the ludicrous, a love of mimicry and a gift for self-deprecation. His poems are riddled with what he termed 'allowable humour', deepening and broadening over the years as the internal heckling voices, the rap-master or banter-king jostle on the page alongside 'pure' lyrical utterance. Hill was 'staggeringly-gifted' as a lyric poet – if in doubt then read again those early poems such as 'Genesis' or 'In Piam Memoriam', and you will come across a young writer with the control and weightiness of visionary utterance to rival Eliot's *Four Quartets* or the best of Edwin Muir or Sidney Keyes. And his doubts concerning such gifts make for the matter of his finest poems:

> Do words make up the majesty
> Of man, and his justice
> Between the stones and the void ?
> > (from 'Three Baroque Meditations')

The doubt here in the punning on 'make up' (constitute or fabricate?) is allowed to resonate; positive and damning readings are allowed to co-exist. Hill's writing is political: he was proud of his working class English origins, a Worcestershire lad, the son of the local bobby, but was revolted by the narrowness of any 'little Englander' approach to culture; his sensibility was European, international. Faith and endurance; attempted heroism and resolve under duress; a fascination with the recurrent and terrible lessons of history; a reverence for the powers of memory; the glories and atrocities of utterance: these are themes explored throughout his poetry from the early nineteen fifties onwards.

Art demands labour at its inception, and demands the same of its audiences: his image of a kindred spirit Ruskin, 'Fellow labouring master-servant' from *The Triumph of Love* is one that embodies Hill's wonderful achievements for me: 'to us he appears/ some half-fabulous field-ditcher who prised/ up, from a stone-wedged hedge-root, the lost/ amazing crown.'

Notes:

[1] For more on Kenneth Curtis, Hill's English teacher at Bromsgrove High School read Norman Rea's moving and elucidatory '9.9.42 Hill, Geoffrey W.', *Agenda*, Vol.30, Nos. 1-2, Spring-Summer 1992.

[2] Originally published in *A Treatise of Civil Power* (Clutag, 2005) this response to Canetti's *Crowds and Power* had parts two and three edited out of the collected poems, *Broken Hierarchies* (OUP, 2015).

[3] From an article in *The North*, Number 44, pp.25-27; ISSN 0269-9885; 2009.

Peter Carpenter

Funeral Music

i.m. Geoffrey Hill

On the morning of your funeral
  in Umbrian heat we slog up our hill
(cragged and steep) heading for Panicale,

to catch our breath in its views back
  over Chiusi and Ceres Lavazza,
my daughter Zoë practising her solo

I Saw The Lord pretty close to pitch
  perfect as we hug any shade going –
our 'Paradiso' an Acqua Frizzante

from the Caffe della Piazza – just to be
  chilling motionless at a table in shade
and studying those black-clothed women

emerging from doorways all economy
  of movement, joining the passing show
of baristas and selfie-takers, and, out of this,

Geoffrey, I wish you eternity away
  from your gallery of dissenters
and dullards, those tongue's atrocities –

so sit you down and rest you here under
  this hand-painted Crucifixion at the base
of the campanile; behind Christ, the sun

striped in gold like Blake's grinning Tyger,
  and you being a boy again who leaps
with serious joy in leaping as I catch the air –

'I saw the Lord sitting on a throne
  High and lifted up   High and lifted up
And his train filled the Temple'

Note:

Zoë was singing *I Saw The Lord*, composed by John Stainer; the opening verse originates in the *Book of Isaiah*, Chapter Six, Verse One, which starts with Isaiah's vision of the Lord's glory: 'In the year that king Uz-zi-ah died I saw also the Lord sitting upon a throne, high and lifted up, and his train filled the temple'. We walked up to Panicale on Monday, 25th July, 2016.

Keith Grant

Geoffrey Hill: a God-given inspiration

I first met Geoffrey Hill through an honorary fellow of Keble College, Oxford, Robin Geffen, who invited me to participate in three annual seminars at the college on the broad theme of creativity in poetry and painting between the Oxford Professor of Poetry and myself, chaired by Robin. The first seminar was titled, 'My Latest Work Is My Best', a notion that most artists would like to apply to themselves. Geoffrey Hill's later work proves beyond doubt the validity of this assertion and his outpouring of thrilling and challenging works in his later life, are for me a God-given inspiration. For me an indispensable aspect of the poetry and critical writings I know of Geoffrey's, apart from its phenomenal reach of scholarship and subject matter, is the balance it achieves between the process and the message in the realisation of its final result. This is for me an inspirational lesson which serves as a profoundly relative example for my own work. During my three annual visits to Keble College I made many portrait sketches of Geoffrey, one of which hangs in the Keble College Senior Common Room, and is one that he particularly admired but said, 'It's magnificent, but you've made me look like King Lear – oh! But I have always wanted to look like Lear!' As I came to know Geoffrey more, a certain professional empathy was established from which I derive great and lasting satisfaction.

On one occasion while we were together walking in the Keble grounds, Geoffrey suddenly asked if I would paint his portrait for the National Portrait Gallery, since they had asked him to nominate an artist. I agreed at once, considering it to be a signal honour even though my life's work as an artist has been more devoted to landscape painting. I determined from the beginning that as well as being a likeness of my sitter, the portrait must refer to Geoffrey Hill's life, his childhood, his family and his art. Most of the imagery in the composition I derived from a memorable visit to his home in Cambridgeshire where I went to make the last drawing study before beginning the painting proper. As I began, Geoffrey enjoined me not to make him look like an old testament prophet – to which he had frequently been likened, nor indeed to make him like King Lear!

The finished painting after months of work was privately unveiled during a dinner hosted by the warden of Keble and Robin Geffen at the college last year. I explained the composition in detail and described most of the imagery. The discerning viewer, however, might want to know the identity of the persons in the three sepia photographs on either side of Geoffrey's head. To the observer's left of my sitter's head is his father in the Khaki uniform of a World War One soldier taken about 1918. To the right of Geoffrey's head is an image of his grandfather in a police inspector's uniform and to the right again is a picture of his great aunt who died of meningitis aged 15 and was a gifted and promising young student artist. All the books are titled legibly and have played a huge part in Geoffrey Hill's creative development. The images like the biplane, the gas-mask and the hour-glass are all to be found in Geoffrey's poetry. The gas-mask and the hour-glass moreover serve also as memento mori. The gas-mask was further inspired by the skull in Holbein's masterpiece, 'The Ambassadors' in the National Gallery, London. Finally, the ghost-like presence of Eric Hosking's barn owl which was used on the dust cover of Hill's slim volume of poetry, 'Clavics', has flown to hover near Geoffrey's left arm in honour of its immortalisation in *Liber Illustrium Virorum*:

The air-treading
Crucifix-pose struck by that
Mousing owl.

Peter Robinson

Balkan Trilogy

In memory of Geoffrey Hill

'prega per Europa'
                    Vittorio Sereni

i

Passport Stamps

There's something about those rock outcrops
along the tops above Dubrovnik,
bloodied, fallen oranges
in the moat around what was Ragusa –
something about a switchback mountain
road that leads inland
(mist rising from a reservoir lake
after temperature-changing rain;
bridge pillars emerging from it
as if from out of nowhere) –
something about an exclamation-mark road sign
when we cross more Dayton borders
and the words
switch back and forth between Roman and Cyrillic –
there's something can't but point towards
past damage, the harms to come...

Nikšić Hotel

Like a convalescent from this month of claim
and counter-claim, I falter
come down to breakfast, seeing as the same
worn carpet would soon alter
when overwhelmed by risen shame
I find no shelter
from the Montenegrin sun's heat, or from casting blame
in a welter
of muffled shouts, disorientation,
hearing news that wrecks it –
plain omelette, bread and tea become
tasteless as the one word *nation*...
Not knowing where to turn for home,
I return to my room through the door marked EXIT.

Herceg Novi

As in a bereavement, when those harms
from your loss are falling
into place with relief at some more evening breeze,
under the prom's transplanted palms
beside seafront concessions
there come, with raucous darts of starlings
at dusk above the old town's eaves,
sensible inward migrations...
so from a balcony, soon after sunrise,
no less at home, you see
spectral headlands jutting to an isolated sea
and can hardly believe your eyes.

Martin Caseley

Geoffrey Hill: A Reading at Aldeburgh, 2009.

A brief recollection.

Around the village of Snape, wooded Suffolk fields and pink pantiled houses give way to a different landscape: gorse bushes fringe the A-roads and a coastal vista of flats spread around the hill. Beyond it, Aldeburgh and the poetry festival. Geoffrey Hill knows this landscape: 'the Alde's thin-ribboned course' and the 'sudden clouds harrowing the Anglian sky' are described in the poem 'Holbein'[1], originally from *'A Treatise of Civil Power'*. I was excited to hear Hill read his work, knowing that he rarely gave public readings and this was a time of a sudden outpouring of his late work, eventually to be published as six volumes of 'The Daybooks'[2].

The two parallel streets of Aldeburgh are not thronged with poetry-lovers, but prosperous groups loiter noisily on the pavements, socialising. An ordinary Saturday afternoon: on the pebbly beach, fishermen sold fresh catches from wooden huts and, within sight of these, the slightly tatty Jubilee Hall awaited. A growing chill reminded me, as the sky dimmed, that it was November.

By ten to four, over 250 people are filling the hall with an expectant undercurrent of talk. On the stage, there are piles of books for sale, drawing browsers. The Aldeburgh Poetry Festival, in its twenty-first year, has done well to attract a writer of Hill's stature. I step aside by the stairs up to the stage to let an old, white-bearded man ascend them tortuously. He takes his time and walks with the aid of a stick, but is appreciative.

Silence at four'o'clock: the introduction reminds the audience of Hill's importance among writers, that he gives very few public readings and makes a request that mobile phones are switched off. Then I get a shock: the old, white-bearded man with a stick shuffles to the microphone – it is Hill!

He wears black and a row of pens in his top pocket; a remembrance poppy is in his lapel; he looks stern, rabbinical, prophetic, but also much older than recent dust jacket pictures.

He reads for 35 minutes, all from unpublished works[3] – a brave and

---

[1] p. 565 , Geoffrey Hill: *Broken Hierarchies: Poems 1952-2013*, edited by Kenneth Haynes (O.U.P, 2013)

[2] All now collected in *Hierarchies*, pp. 625 – 936.

[3] This piece was originally drafted in 2009, when most of *The Daybooks* had not been published.

demanding appeal to the loyalty of his readers. There is material from a sequence inspired by Donatello's sculpture 'Habakkuk', which Hill came face to face with in Rome[4], and also pieces from a sequence of madrigals, inspired by Tippett's 1952 'Dance, Clarion Air'. Other sequences are in Sapphic meter or connected with the life of Aneurin 'Nye' Bevin, which Hill introduces by speaking admiringly of Michael Foot's autobiography.[5] The audience are enthralled and respectful, and Hill reads with complete stentorian authority, keen to emphasise rhythms and form, even jokingly offering to beat out the stresses of a line with his stick. This is of a part with the sly undercurrent of dry humour in Hill's introductions – something long-time readers will be familiar with – and at one point, a smattering of spontaneous clapping wrongfoots him, and he has to have it explained as 'appreciation'.

After the allotted thirty-five minutes he stops, to great applause. A queue quickly forms when he agrees to sign books; there is a frisson of astonishment at this. He sits onstage signing and chatting, crouched at a desk, a Blakean, Old Testament figure, leavened with dry, sardonic notes. Outside the light fades beyond the beach of pebbles.

---

[4] See *Al Tempo De' Tremuoti*, *The Daybooks VI*, sections 22 and 40, pp. 896, 906, *Hierarchies*.
[5] The 'Nye' references are in 'Oraclau' *The Daybooks III*, sections 62 – 67, pp. 761 – 763, *Hierarchies*.

Omar Sabbagh

His Solitude

Geoffrey Hill, RIP

There's a tall, burly wall between
Loneliness and solitude.

He spoke

Peerlessly through his palace,
A man bold enough to be
Lean and tortured,
Echoing

In a gilded hall of echoes
A speech that verged and cusped for
The parley of a host
Of very different mirrors –

More grand than grandiose.

He was canny as the snake, footless
With his bone-sunken feet –
His marrow to his bone now's
Seamless, sewn, narrow and neat.

So let the animals roar: their
Mulching school begins no more –

As one sage goes sagely through the door
To a different place,
A better,

Reflector now of reflector.

Peter Dale

Two Anecdotes

When I worked on *Agenda* I had several brief meetings with Geoffrey Hill. Dates and places escape me these days but one was before we gave a reading at the Cockpit Theatre in London. We met in a pub beforehand: Geoffrey, Michael Hamburger and John Heath-Stubbs. The first two were there when I arrived but were not on speaking terms over some recent dispute and I, the hapless rookie, struggled to make conversation. Then the street door was flung open and John, partially sighted, blundered in, heading straight ahead to where he thought the bar was, disarranging tables and chairs. This did not break the deadlock between the two first arrivals but at least helped me out a bit.

On a later more relaxed and interesting occasion, we met in William Cookson's flat. The conversation came round to the mysterious effect some buildings and places have on people that are moved by them malignly or benignly. I mentioned how William, in our college days, had wanted to show me the Epstein statue in one of the quads. I had astounded William by refusing to enter it, saying it overpowered me with a feeling of evil. Geoffrey responded with a similar experience, saying a friend let him use his cottage when he was working on a poem but after a day or so he had to leave because the cottage affected him with an oppressive feeling of evil.

Andrew McNeillie

Visiting Again

I had to follow up. Not to would be wrong.
And so I phoned to ask him over.
'Afraid I can't take bus-rides any more,' he said.
'They knock the stuffing out of me.
It's very kind of you... But if you'd like
to drop by for a bite and take pot luck –
what my wife used to call a "non-lunch" –
with a glass of red: please come along'...

The polar opposites of selfhood –
duty versus the detached and private life –
can cross and spark, if all too rarely,
like the moment of a poem itself.
Take things as they come, I counselled.
Think what it must be like to grow old...
Like a back number in a waiting room,
faded and more than slightly foxed.

'Believe me, they know not what they say,
when they say it's the thought that counts.'
The first thing he said as we sat down.
He picked at his food with little appetite.
I asked how it'd been when he started out.
'You might wonder. How long have you got?
Do I remember?' he paused. 'I suppose:
to hear the pentameter, *that* was the first heave.'

He winked and leaning forward topped us up.
'Not all bad this screwtop stuff, d'you think?'...
Then: 'To MAKE IT TRUE ...' he proclaimed.
'MAKE IT TRUE ... true to nature,
to the eye's window on the world out there.
What else?' He stared at the bottle, distracted
a while, as if contemplating options,
or else far-distant planetary systems.

'I mean true to the heart's workings,
hardest of all to find a language for.
Then do the police... as the man said.
Find your voice discovering voices.
Remember our greatest poet was a ventriloquist.'
I caught his eye. 'I *mean* Shakespeare, of course.
Then history in all its glory and lapses,
the curse of quislings of all descriptions...

'(you know poetry's no stranger to those).
The magic there is in words and rhyming:
oh ever-after leave, and ever-after stay.
Rhythm that chimes. But it's the thought...
I *don't* mean sincerity. That's something else.
Of course there's no such thing as "pure" poetry.
Pure of what, I want to know?
No intention whatever! Pure of the reader?

'Don't give me "poetry for poetry's sake"...
For life's sake, surely, for delight and thought,
solitude, contemplation, melancholy,
cathartic sorrow; and the scourge of folly –
the craft itself since time began. Forget
that priesthood beyond fen causeway
with nothing to say but how to say nothing,
word-play impervious to sense as geese to rain.'

Eye razed an I, brow beaten, straitfaced,
words-in-thwart thwart-in-words:
REVOLUTION this way that way chased
freeze of epic vase held siege. I thought.
But not a ha'penny for theme. Wood give me,
dark odd to sea useless. Waking, swiftly said:
'All poets make a virtue of what they do
as if they had much say in the matter'...

'Anything goes these days,' he rattled on.
'Declare yourself a poet and that'll do:
you'll be a fraud in residence tomorrow.
Can you imagine a *Spirit of the Age* now?
Can't you hear Hazlitt spinning in his grave?
I hear they call it the post-literary era.
"Intrinsic value: Rest in Peace"... our epitaph.
Either way, there is no *zeitgeist* anymore'...

He'd seen no one else all week, barring
the Ocado man; and he was stir crazy,
under the siege only death can raise.
Now he fell silent and seemed melancholy.
Next he got up, crossed to the window,
glass in hand, and peered out into
his own reflection, saying as he did:
'Some things must be believed to be seen'...

'And how's *your* work coming along?'
'Oh, you know how it is.' He shrugged.
'Well, perhaps I do'... '*Plus ça change*,' I said,
though to whom now seemed unclear.
'But... while I remember, I wanted you to hear this.'
He waved a CD: '"The Leningrad",
USSR State Symphony, 1962 – that stickler
Konstantin Ivanov in command...

'So much of that era, those darkest days.'
And as he put it on, quite out of nowhere:
'I suppose you saw my dear friend died
the other day?... Leaving me the last of us.
I told him he must *not* predecease me. But
there we are. I couldn't make it all that way
to pay my respects in person. So upsetting
and a shame, I like a poet's funeral best of all'...

He sat back a while and settled in to listen,
then as the *danse macabre* ended
just as the poignant third began,
something rattled his cage and he was off again.
'You know you'll have to do your bit at mine,
write me up in *The Times*? (Be sure you scotch
those rumours I was once a spy.) Pull out
the stops. But *no* organ music of any kind.

'And no dog-collared eulogy. My daughter
knows the score. I've told her about you.'
An old man's vanity is as hard to bear as any...
'What *do* we mean by personal tragedy?'
He threw out suddenly, and answered at once,
'Something more than mere mortality.
"Ten Days that Shook the World" maybe,
the torments of *King Lear* – not just growing old.

'Age walks hand-in-hand with irrelevance,
each the other's under-study, you know?
The sorry truth that haunts backstage
as the audience raises the roof on a rising star –
to boost the latest Hamlet's bungled grief.'
At last I pulled myself up from my chair.
'I'm sorry,' he said, 'I spend too much time alone.
Thank you for coming. Age is a nightmare

'I struggle to wake from. I need a guide.
I need someone to lead me back to light,
a Virgil or a Beatrice if you like'...
I walked home, rehearsing my speech as I went,
while all about the rush-hour gridlocked –
the evening, unearthly, hung in clouds of exhaust
and frailer breath, as the temperature plummeted
as if towards Leningrad itself.

Note:
The old poet in this poem is not Geoffrey Hill, nor his visitor Andrew McNeillie.

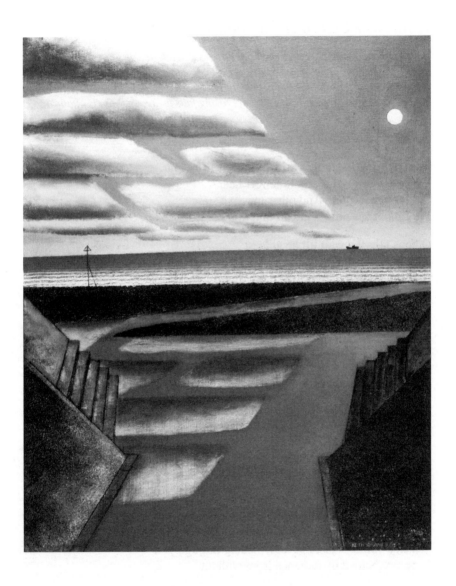

Rainer Maria Rilke

From *Neue Gedichter* (In Rodin's Garden)

*'I have gone through countless cycles of birth and death, seeking but not
finding the builder of this house which is my body. How painful are birth
and death again and again! But now that I have seen you, house-builder, you shall
not build my house again. Every kind of craving falls away: nirvana is attained.'*

Dhammapada, 153, 154

Buddha ('Als ob er horchte')

As if he were listening. Stillness: as if from afar...
We go our way, and can no longer hear.
He, though, is star. And other massive stars
We cannot see now stand around him here.

O he is all. We wait till he at least
Notices us. But does he, really, need to?
And if we knelt to him, whom all things kneel to,
He'd stay inert, as deep as stone or beast.

For that which here now at his feet compels us
To fall evolved in him light-years ago.
And he forgets the only things we know,
And what he thinks and knows expels us.

Buddha in Glory

Centre of all centres, core of cores,
Almond, self-enclosing and self-sweetening,
All we see beneath the circling stars
Is your fruit-flesh: hear our prayer – our greeting –

You who feel now nothing clinging to you,
And whose house is *in* the Infinite,
Whence strong saps arise and, pulsing through you
Here, are helped by radiance from without.

For, above you, all your suns,
Full and glowing, turn: you turn them –
While, within, what now begins
Will outlive, outburn them.

At Rilke's Grave

… 'This time the examination showed that he had leukaemia in a rare and especially painful form that first manifests itself in the intestines and in the final stage produces black pustules on the mucous membranes of the mouth and nose. These burst and bleed, making it difficult for the patient to drink, so that he is plagued by thirst as well as unremitting pain.'

W. Leppmann, *Rilke: A Life*

Rose, oh reiner Widerspruch, Lust,
Niemandes Schlaf zu sein unter soviel
Lidern.

*

Rilke's Last Poem – Sanatorium Val-Mont, December 1926

Come then, you last – incurable – amazing
Torment: I feel you spreading through my body.
I blazed in spirit – whereas now I'm blazing
In you. The wood resisted, but is ready
To accept your flames now – cease to try to quell
You – feed your furious presence – nurture you.
My earthly mildness turns to a final hell
Of pain, like fire which has no then – no now.
Free of all futures, planless, and quite pure,
I have ascended this chaotic pyre,
Certain that nowhere, for my hoarding heart –
Now silenced – can a future still be bought.
Is it still I who burn? No memory shows me
Who I once was. Fire turns all memories
To ash. O life, o life – outside of this.
And I in raging flame. Here no one knows me.

*

Consumed at last by pain like fire, Rilke composed for his own or any gravestone:

Rose, oh pure contradiction, desire
To be no one's sleep under so many
Eyelids.

Translated by W D Jackson

Note:

Rilke's gravestone (in Raron, high above the Rhone valley) bears only his name and epitaph. The epitaph (quoted and translated in the poem) was written and included by Rilke in his will in October 1925, when he was already seriously ill. Rilke's last poem, *Komm du, du letzter*, was found in his notebook after his death on 29 December, 1926.

Rainer Maria Rilke

You, lost in advance

You, lost in advance
beloved, the one who never arrived,
what sounds you love most I cannot say.
No more do I seek, in the moment's surging wave
to know you. All the great images in me,
the deep felt distant landscape,
cities and towers and bridges and
unexpected turns in the path
and those mighty lands
through which Gods once passed
raise within the certainty
of you eluding me.

Alas, gardens you are,
my gaze lingered over with such
hope. An open window
in the country-house, you almost stepping out
pensive to greet me. Lanes I came upon –
that you had just passed down,
and sometimes the mirrors of the shops
were still dizzy with you and startled
gave back my own too sudden image – who knows,
if the same bird did not call through both of us
yesterday, alone, in the evening?

Translated by Will Stone

From *Poems 1910 to 1922* (Paris, Winter 1913/14)

Carol Rumens

Collection Plate

I picked up all the balls of silver paper
that had once been sweets and put them in the coconut shell
where birds once fed: it was a useless gesture.
The people-smuggler Chaeron makes our souls wait and wait
and they think his horrible little dinghy's heaven,
and they ply him with cash and gifts, and even give him their daughters.
The screaming of the terrified girls mingles
with the howling and crying of those who've nothing to sell,
not even a little ball of silver paper.

Nant y Garth

i.m. Yuri Drobyshev

As the bus wound its way up Nant y Garth
it was as if the birchwoods either side
were gathering height. I heard their
choirs amassing light: bass, tenor, alto,
soprano, entering one by one, like green
combers, cliffs of melody, with depths
and peaks I couldn't fully sense, but knew
sang gladness – gladness of the wakened branches,
and peeled buds, and leaves called to the sun
for the first time, to stream into their year –
no, their much-less-than year – of darkening grace.
I could no more believe the sap insensible,
than I believe the dead are broken branches,
and all their self-songs censored or extinguished.

Angela Readman

The Crows Invite Us to Grieve

The sky is an invitation to grieve,
as I cart out the morning in plastic sacks.

Crows on the wall plot their ink, craw
to a dead bird displaying rain on the lawn,

snapped beads. It starts with one beak
pinning a stick to a cold leg, arrows

of fern on a breast, buds of a dandelion
I casually pulled. And suddenly the sky

is winged wild, the pale cotton of day
scorched by bird after bird arcing

the path of sorrow above us, delivering
a eulogy in voices that can't carry a tune.

Outside, I listen to scraps of murder fly
out of mouths, a silk nightdress falls

out of my bag, the scent of lemon
bath oil, straps of *When I Fall in Love,*

spill a lifetime of overheard songs,
half sung, all over the sun-spattered path.

The Bees Sing Our Night Songs

The drone of the ceiling fan slices our silence.
Mother stares at the bed, so many small deaths
on her face, always. The bee on the window

wanders star to star, separate to the drift,
drunk on the lilies in the vase. I cup it in palms
full of unclosed amens to carry outside.

The sky is dusted in a pollen of stars, dark,
light, as country preacher's robe under glass.
Every lamp in the house blares, air laden

with my father's breath, my mother's hope
to decipher a sermon, sorry, love from a gasp.
She is firmly inside, I am out. Bee in hand,

a quaker's velvet on my skin, I place the insect
on the rough wooden hive, a whole night on its back,
white-wash sawing the moonlight into laths.

I stare at the house. The hive purrs a eulogy
to the pruned roses as I wait for curtains to close
and mouth the news. Tonight, I start to live.

Gill McEvoy

Growth Rings

Once she was willow, her narrow skirt
a strip of sunlight in the woodland,
her blouse an unfurled leaf.

As maple she wore skirts of scarlet,
fretted sleeves
that showed her skin like clouds.

Now oak.
Jackets of knubble and gnarl.
Thickening, thickening.

Acorns at her feet.

In Red and White

You could helter-skelter down their columns on a rug or tray,
pretend they're giant sticks of rock in red and white –

slice through their middles and you'd surely find
the names of places where they stand:
Strumble, Needles, Bardsey, Portland Bill.

In the wind you hear the thin bewildered sighs
of long-forgotten keepers who drift round
the eerie robot systems that transmit the beams;
men amazed that no-one has to trim or light the lamps.

Seán Street

Mozart's Starling

Mozart bought a pet starling on 27 May 1784.
When it died, on 4 June, 1787, he gave the bird
a funeral.

Before, I was only one of a flock
touching down in broken buildings,
and perhaps life is a quaver
in this duet we make together,
but teach me your song and I
will extemporize upon it a while.

While you cage my voice I catch yours,
 a mutual loving belonging
with no method or meaning in it
except what we make in partnership,
another music, a shared
predicament in our patterns of living.

I see that you weep because you cannot fly,
and I sob my sounds because
you will not free me.

                    As sunsets grow frantic
with song, I tense for stillness
to preserve mine for dawn, you and I
both parts of the same brief melody,
my oiled wing and your laughing sadness,
with nowhere else anything left
but silence. What better brotherhood is there,
that you hear my trapped crying
while I imitate yours? There's no existence
but to be part of a whole
shared being.

I have no complaint
if you steal my song from me,
because I will die with yours in my throat.
So play for me Amadeus
and I will answer, brothers now
in the moment. A symphony starts with
one note, so let us sing a while,
then bury me as befits a minstrel.

Jeremy Hooker

Greenfinches

Convalescing,
you stood by the window
delighting to watch them –
parent birds flying
from tree to garden hedge,
fledglings trembling
on the verge of flight.

How free they seemed –
quick-winged, filling the air
with moss-green,
a flash of yellow,
a dash of song.

How they flourish,
you thought, how free –
until this:
two young ones
dead, necks broken
against the glass.

Here, at this big window,
which lets in the light,
the healing light, where
you have looked out, feeling
on imprisoning days something
within you that could almost fly.

The Green Woodpecker

There is nostalgia
that draws me back
into the mire, and there is love
that liberates.

So I call on you to guide me
bird of the laughing call
greenback, redhead
with yellow rump.

How laboured
your flight seems,
looping from grove to glade
anthill to anthill
as if you would fall.

Did you fly into the painted cave
or out of it – bird
on a stick in the shaman's hand?

Old one, you were always
most at home on the ground
beak ploughing
for larvae and ants.

Yet nostalgia
also can be an energy –
memory a flight
that gives wings to the mind.

My father
was a gardener and a painter
but no bird-man.

Once, in the greenhouse
he found, wings beating
wildly among tomatoes
in peaty warmth,
what he thought a parrot.

And indeed there is
something exotic
about you, native bird.

Yaffle,
yaffingale
of ancient times
woodpecker
'who also is Zeus'
rain-bird
thunder-spirit
from how far back
you fly into our world.

From glade to grove,
from anthill to anthill,
you fly –
no drummer of dead wood
but a bird with a beak
for digging, a soil-grubber
since Mars was a farmer.

And why do I call you now,
in age the boy I was
relishing my short time,
laughing one,
greenback in the green wood?

Here I come
with scratched legs
from heath to cover
of the ancient trees,
and there you are
looping from glade to grove

as if you would fall.

Blackthorn and Celandine

Anticipation's the word.

Snatches of song from birds
remembering to sing,
voices coming back...
Pairings, skirmishes –
a new thought in wintry air,
a spirit waking.

I wait for the first white tuft,
a snowflake of flower
on the black bough,
a feathering
before the touch of green.
I look in ditch and on hedge-bank
for a yellow star,
first of a constellation.

And now there's no sign,
only a feeling, a memory.

Other years pile up,
leaves on leaves, a mould
that accumulates,
a weight on the heart,
a burden on the mind.

And what is this
but something to grow in,
compost for a green shoot?

'Old man', you say,
surprised, as if coming awake.

You think of the world
you have not changed;
you dream of the lives
you've dreamed of,
possibilities unrealised;
you see the very globe,
the folly of the kind you are.

And so you wait, watching
for the first white tuft
against the black bough,
anticipating the first yellow star.

What's new, old man?

It's always the same,
this newness,
and you are ever in love with it,

eager for what may come.

Peter McDonald

Weaveley Furze

for G H, on leaving his Chair, 2015

So: to keep going on the glum route-march,
a mile's trudge in the summer across fields
where either a dropped match
or the farmer on purpose burned the crop
crisp black; or else sunshine, that nothing shields
us from; or else dumb mischief; till we stop
at a thin gate with a rope latch
fraying from the top.

The Glyme and the Dorn, not even half-full
are not so much as half heard, yet the trees
make their leaves voluble
as they shush like a river overhead.
Down here, sticky brambles and homebound bees
inheriting their commonwealths, instead
of this binding, unenforceable
contract with the dead

which no one can believe in any more,
spread at their own speeds; now at your deaf side
I lessen the uproar
but can't pretend the noise has gone away.
Someone has cut logs into sticks, and tied
them in faggots, and left them: you could say
they're sound, or rotten at the core,
mugging pure dismay:

ghastly, ghastly. Maybe it's just the heat,
or the staginess of advancing years,
but the young do seem to bleat
(I'm younger; I'm not young) a deadly din
round and about us now while, *unawares*,
something expires. Still there's nothing to win:
the courage, just, to leave your seat,
take breath, and begin.

Newcastle Island, British Columbia 2015

for Alan and Philippa Southgate

Our best steps are the steps we take
on purpose, and just for the sake
of knowing they will bring us here:
from a ferry to a landing-pier,
from one room to another room,
or from two countries to one home
with no location maps can give,
but where we know we have to live.
Two lives can even step across
the line that each knows how to gloss
as a threshold only they can see
into the place that has to be,
where everything is as it was
and yet completely changed, because
its west is east, below above,
and love and love are the one love.

The tricks of time are nothing much:
for if I am not here as such,
it's only a few weeks ago
that I went on the short and slow
trip to a place I want to make
over to you for its own sake.
Newcastle Island, off the coast
not far from here, I'll give to you
as land that I myself came to
for only a day, and somehow
for ever; where the tides allow
flat rock to dry beneath huge trees,
and birds and beasts go as they please
on ways they know, unknown to us,
without decision, without fuss;
the sunshine on Kanaka Bay
for one hour never can give way
to cloud or shadows or dark night;
the purple martins in their flight
are buoyant for eternity
over a cold and flashing sea.

No more than ten minutes afloat,
only a short step off the boat
and here you are, for now you've crossed
where nothing ever can be lost
entirely, and the silence sounds
through seas and forests with no bounds
as entire lifetimes come and go.
The best thing of us that we know
we cross into, invisibly,
a threshold we can only see
together, for when we're alone
there's nothing truly seen or known;
but here it is, and here you are,
as far is near, and near is far:
love, the one place we travel to,
for ever somehow, here with you.

Louis Aragon

I think of you Robert (Desnos)

Your voice was charged with something of Nerval
You spoke of blood most singular young man
Your cruel formal verse you made it scan
Laughter of butchers flanked you in Les Halles
You seemed already to be laying odds
Across the years I hear the resonance
Poetic tyro slaughtered in advance
Avenged back then by sneers at men and gods

You left Compiègne I think of you Robert
Just as asleep one evening you had said
So you fulfilled that prophecy you made
Fate of our century lies bleeding there

Stood in a doorway with a twist of fries
St Merry overhung by thunderclouds
Impertinently staring down the crowds
You gazed like royal-blood Nereides
Enormous throbbing with a pallid haze
Ground at your foot like foam at breast of nude
Thick with fag-ends and cabbage chewed and spewed
Footfall of rain and all-too-ready lays

You left Compiègne I think of you Robert
Just as asleep one evening you had said
So you fulfilled that prophecy you made
Fate of our century lies bleeding there

It's you it still is you still strolling on
Shepherd of long desires dead reveries
The Champs-Elysées dim below the trees
Until your own domain the night is gone
Oh Gare de l'Est first croissant of the day
Black coffee percolated freshly poured
Crisp morning papers pungent boulevard
The metro-mouths where figures drained away

You left Compiègne I think of you Robert
Just as asleep one evening you had said
So you fulfilled that prophecy you made
Fate of our century lies bleeding there

Your passing haunts the city's grimy brows
With coloured shade   The Sacré-Cœur is wan
As knacker daybreak flays the Pantheon
With shreds and tatters   Later in the Bois
The sun rolls oranges itself an orange
The moon transfers her seat from tower to tower
Striking the belfries as they strike the hour
And the wind howls beneath the Pont-au-Change

You left Compiègne I think of you Robert
Just as asleep one evening you had said
So you fulfilled that prophecy you made
Fate of our century lies bleeding there

Translated by Timothy Adès

Graham Hardie

The sea of Eden's garden

come adrift with my sad muse, let me feel
your anxiety, the stifling of your sexuality;
come adrift with me, let us sail on the massive
sea of Eden's garden, a love unrequited in fashion,
but felt by those on bended knee; let the waves be naked,
as I see your flesh in the heart's imagination, the ripple
of breast and the poignancy of possession;
let me see the shells of your tears and the animosity
of your fears, as we abandon the notions of all that is given
by the treacherous motion of what we believe and see!
and let me slide by the mast, the wooden, selfish incantation
of your soul, hardened by grief and mortuary and blank
with the face of celibacy.

David Pollard

Rodrigo at the Keyboard

The keyboard fingered
white to the touch and black
in the mind's braille
and counterpoint to sound's
own world of meaning and detachment;
each key, a sliver of sight's silence,
has its colour, vivid as juniper and magic,
mapping another conscience of vibrations
in the air and time.

And just above a quaver,
somewhere in the visible
of a deathbed lay the body of love,
his love in its last notations of decay
that his musicianship will never fever back
into tonality.

Fingertip, tender as creation, roams
along the curves and dips
of its lost strumming, tensions,
hesitations of the muse
pluck at its pizzicatos and vibrations
chordal with its own polyphony
he knew and simply,
quietly,
in the distance of its loneliness,
drew forth.

A Virginall

Oh I have plucked her, tongued her white ivories
against the air, Dowland I think it was, October
winding the chordal branches of her soundings
twined into subtle modulations of high breeding.

Yet I demanded more. She was too painted,
inlay too delicate for my fingerings;
piano to my forte, her flavour fading at the touch,
her limbs almost too faint to hold the dance.

She was too gentle for my temperings,
feathered with beauty of the retiring kind,
the play of quill making faint counterpoint
to lie upon the air of her nobility.

A Tenth Pavanne she did with me
slow as the fire in human veins allowed
in duple metre as the custom is, then
fell into her rest of broken heartstrings

and too many splintered
bones of other longings.

Jeremy Page

Leaving

They are leaving.

Soon the house will have forgotten
the rhythm of their days.
It will no longer witness
their early morning rising,
the comings and goings
that have punctuated their lives.

It will not know those evenings
in dead of winter
when the lights they read by
were the only lights for miles.

And all they will take away
are memories – half forgotten
visits, wedding breakfasts
for marriages long dissolved,
good times, bad, indifferent –
the missing pieces
of the jigsaw they leave behind.

When I left for the last time
I had no reason to suppose
that I would never return,
so I cannot imagine
how it will feel to drive away
along the lane so often driven –
nor how they will now look back.

Elizabeth Barton

Now You're Back

You've been away so long
I've missed your shoes shucked
in the hall, the feel of cool cotton
beneath my fingers as I iron
your shirts. Steam mists
my eyes as the soleplate glides
like skates on ice, leaping chasms,
thawing snow-capped peaks.

I wish we could smooth the rucks
of our love, repair the seam we've ripped.

The iron sighs, bonds
loosening, as I search for you
in the nooks of gauntlets, cuffs,
roam the salt-bleached wastes
of yoke and tail. I press
so hard, the light shines through
and the cloth feels almost
as warm as your skin.

Swallowtail

I have no net to catch you
no setting board, no insect pin.

I know you will come: the garden glows
with the fruits of passion flowers, pots of red hibiscus.
Beyond the dirt road is a farm where pigs loaf beneath the olive trees,
orchards of almond and fig. Clouds slip away; in a dazzle of sun I see you
hurling yourself over the roof tiles, down to the lavender beds
as though you know this sweetness cannot last.

You pause on a cluster of red sage
your wings so huge they make the blood moon tremble.
I hold my breath as I glimpse colours bright as eternity, yellow wings
chequered with black, as playful as the Jack of Spades,
a mirror image of itself with its red and blue
false eyes, tails delicate as silken thread

and you fling yourself
into the frayed web of my heart.

Dylan Jones

Acres

When I was young
I'm sure my mother must have said

look – life has a thousand acres
and they are filled with worry and noise –

but perhaps I'm imagining things –
perhaps it was me who did the filling –

And now I wish
I had emptied the green fields
of the fear that poured through me
because, winding through the rye grass
and winding through the wheat
is the one path – whatever

And surely the easiest expression
sees the lips bend
into a smile

And the best option
surely is to square up,
face the badness when it comes
not weeks, months, years
ahead
of what might never be

And it's good
the eyes lift sometime,
face the sky,
be it sun, or bird, or stars
that are dancing there

When I was young
I should have told my father
told my mother

life is eaten up with waste
do not shadow the good seed

Cat's Ears

And I think of my mother
again, after many days
and weeks when I moved
happily in her absence.
It was the cat
who prompted her memory –
the way he washed his ears,
the paws flicking across them
in a vigorous sweep –

'It's going to rain'
she would say,
'the cat's washing
his ears right over.'
And I would laugh –

the morning sun
spotted the white
net curtains
with shadow and light –

birds on the lawn
bickered among
the bread and scraps
my mother had scattered –

But by mid-afternoon
the sky had thickened with grey,
and a thin drizzle lowered itself
slowly masking the elm-tops –

And the cat
watched the wet
empty lawn
through the closed French window –

And my mother
hummed the happy air
of *I told you so!*

David Attwooll

Otmoor

i

a tightening tide felt
   here in the country's navel
      a hundred miles from the sea

no hierarchy of land
   and water   compounded
      indeterminate wetland

the landscape inverts
   subject   object
      seeps into language

light skids off a ditch
   in a brisk wind
      a flit   a marshy hollow

a pill   quaking bog
   in the old course
      the River Ray misses

blurred calligraphy   reeds
   layering of sedges
      rushes   coarse grass

a kind of openness
   something gone away
      brought back again

ii

at the moor's edge
a red-eyed radio mast
the hill's exclamation
broadcasts through space

near the moor's hub
a huge ammonite lies in the mud
her spiral has listened to time
for sixty million years

iii

waterbirds rehearse
their repertoire of impressions:

felt mallets
striking a marimba

ricochets from a 50's
cowboy shoot-out

small waves scuffing
a wooden hull

the sound of a pattern
intricate and oriental

chatter of circling stars
in daytime when no-one sees

W S Milne

Torry

The foghorn at Girdle Ness,
   Margaret, remember?
The deep-throated thunder of the surf
desolate at dusk, in the gloaming,
restless as our own thoughts?
The north wind battering the sea-wall,
fields burnt with sea-spray,
plovers wheeping the air?
The kirk that stood on the headland
with trawlers as backdrop –
   retreating horizons,
                   time's drift,
the cliffs that fall away,
   breakers forever breaking,
the years that cannot stay.

Angela Kirby

The Railings

Unpainted for years, rusting through the Depression
and the war, those that hemmed our fields by now were
twisted here and there; bent perhaps by a panicked rush
of shorthorns, a carelessly driven hay cart or by one
of the great horses easing a fly-stung itch on its vast rump
yet with their lower bars misted by Queen Anne's lace,
Ragged Robin and mayflowers, they still kept something
of their style, a hint of past elegance which pleased us.
Look, just here, this stretch by the hawthorn tree is where
we practised our vaults in the long summers, tasting
the thrills of take-off, that dream-sense of flying, while
over there, between the upper and lower fields, bored
with the ease and predictability of homemade jumps,
we'd set the horses at the metal fence, Beautiful Charlotte,
Boy, Jonathan and Bracken collected into rocking-horse
canters, then urged on till we were soaring up and over,
careless of entanglement and the intransigence of iron.

Thunder

God's moving his furniture again,
she said, every time it thundered
and would take to the cupboard
under the stairs with her favourite
blue rosary beads and a yellowing
stump of holy candle which had
wept for years. Father pointed out
with unanswerable Protestant logic
that we were far more likely to die
by the candle setting fire to all those
old newspapers she'd stored there
than by any lightning strikes; still
she prayed for him, sure that his
conversion was at even longer odds.

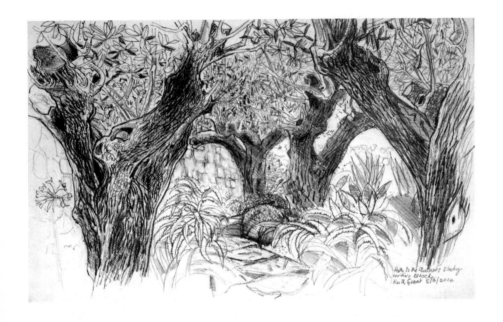

Path to the Author's Study,
verdure block,
Keith Grant 5/8/2014

John Robert Lee

The Sacred in Poetry

Contributing to a symposium, *Faith that illuminates* (1935), T.S. Eliot, in a presentation titled 'Religion and Literature' said: 'The whole of modern literature is corrupted by what I call Secularism, that it is simply unaware of, simply cannot understand the meaning of, the primacy of the supernatural over the natural life'. Proposing that 'the "greatness" of literature cannot be determined solely by literary standards,' he suggested that 'literary criticism should be completed by criticism from a definite ethical and theological standpoint.'

Leon Wieseltier, reviewing Czeslaw Milosz's *The Witness of Poetry* in 1983 in *The New Republic*, quotes Milosz's question to the Harvard audience for his Charles Eliot Norton lectures: 'Is non-eschatological poetry possible?' Those lectures were published in the book, and Wieseltier, in his review, noted 'Milosz's insistence upon a dimension of the holy is its appositeness to the age.' For the reviewer, Milosz's 'solution is the resacralization of the world.' And the author himself asks, in the first essay, 'How did it happen that to be a poet of the twentieth century means to receive training in every kind of pessimism, sarcasm, bitterness, doubt?'

In what seems the domineering secularism of our time, one can find many important representative voices like Eliot's and Milosz's and Geoffrey Hill's, making the case for the sacred and sacramental in our modern literatures. While one can find writers with similar concerns in other cultures, I am reflecting in a general way on Western contemporary writers of the recent past, who have raised the banners of faith and imagination against the all-pervasive pressures of a technologized, materialistic age.

Gregory Wolfe, the American editor and founder of *Image: A Journal of the Arts and Religion*, has recorded in his book of essays *Intruding upon the timeless (2003)* how the Journal was born. As he puts it, for many, 'the secular master narratives, such as Marxism and Freudianism had failed to live up to their initial promise... they left their adherents unable to account for the true wellsprings of good and evil.' He noted that a hunger had grown, 'for a deeper understanding of mystery, that borderland where reason fails and only faith and imagination can go.' What Wolfe and his colleagues discovered on launching the magazine (against their fears and doubts) was that 'our interest in the intersection between faith and imagination was shared by myriad artists and writers all over the world.' They were not interested in an image that existed in a 'sort of self-imposed religious ghetto... but had to be present on the public square... for it is precisely in the imaginative space created by works of art that a diverse, multicultural society can explore religious matters without the divisiveness of polemics and propositions... into this fragmented and contentious world, art that engages faith can body forth an incarnational balance between the letter and the spirit, make ancient truths new, and allow the time-bound to briefly and tentatively intrude upon the timeless.'

For those seeking a fresh grounding (or perhaps a starting point) to understand the importance and place of the sacred in our lives, Philip Sherrard's *The Sacred in Life and Art* (1990) provides a well-wrought beginning. 'The very idea of the sacred presupposes to start with the presence of the Divine or the existence of God. Without the Divine – without God – there can be no holiness, nothing sacred.' Gerard Manley Hopkins, in whose work the sacred rests in both the celebratory cry and in dark soul anguish, sings out:

The world is charged with the grandeur of God.
It will flame out, like shining from shook foil

To manifest the sacred in poetry and to propose its centrality in our secular world is to raise the Divine against all that denies it. Sherrard writes, ' the concept of a completely profane world – of a cosmos wholly desacralized – is a fairly recent invention of the human mind... the presence of God... is the initial and ultimately unique presupposition of the sacred, for the simple reason that without that presence there is no sacredness anywhere... the first symptom of the profane mind – of the idolatrous mind – is its habit of separating its ideas of things from the idea of God...[and] you have set out on the path that leads to the desacralization... of the things themselves.'

For Sherrard, 'the theme of the transcendent' is crucial to the understanding of the sacred. Many holistic approaches often leave out the transcendent, focusing only on the psychological and physical realms. Poetry that reflects the sacred recognizes, in Sherrard's words, 'without participation in God there can be no escaping fragmentation, disintegration, self-alienation, however much we may struggle against them.' And have these not been and still are, distinguishing themes and anxieties of much of our literature for the past century and this one?

On a personal note: it was an epiphanic moment for me, years ago now gone out of memory, when I discovered Francis Thompson's poem 'The Kingdom of God'. While I was then far from formulating concepts of the sacramental or the sacred in poetry, I was moved by and somehow never forgot, these lines:

... upon thy so sore loss
Shall shine the traffic of Jacob's ladder
Pitched betwixt Heaven and Charing Cross.
... And lo, Christ walking on the water
Not of Gennesareth, but Thames.

Ok, so I am a Caribbean person, living most of my life in my small island St. Lucia. But in the words of Nobel laureate Derek Walcott, I benefited from a 'sound colonial education,' and these names out of Imperial Central London were familiar. I struggle to recall, but I know what caught my attention was that bold juxtaposition of Heaven and Charing Cross, of Gennesareth and Thames. Here, through some dim and barely recognized perception, I was pointed to the transcendent, the immanent, the Divine in the mix of the madding crowd and our most mundane activities.

Of course Thompson's poem is about that:

O world invisible, we view thee,
O world intangible, we touch thee,
O world unknowable, we know thee,
Inapprehensible, we clutch thee!

And he speaks of the naturalness of the inevitable communion of the sacred and the earthy. The drift of angels' wings, 'beats at our own clay-shuttered doors'. So close are they that, 'Turn but a stone, and start a wing!' The sacred is among us, and available, but it is our indifferent, careless, agnostic hearts, 'that miss the many-splendoured thing'. And so he celebrates, he exalts, he boldly affirms the sacred, comforting presences at Charing Cross and the Thames, travelling graciously with us in our own mind-darkened ('benumbed conceiving') concrete jungles.

I think now that this poem of Thompson's was growing its influence deep in the subconscious when I came to write *Canticles*, poems that planted the sacred and transcendent in the named streets of my capital Castries, on the beaches, in the hills of my native island home St. Lucia. Using images from folk music – its instruments and dances, traditional dress, the Kwéyòl language – as well as contemporary reggae music, international news headlines and so on – I wrote poems that I have described as a 'Caribbean Pilgrim's Progress'. Poems of faith rooted in the milieu of flesh and blood reality. Other influences have certainly been Donne and Herbert, Hopkins and Eliot and a host of other modern Caribbean writers like Derek Walcott, Kamau Brathwaite, Lorna Goodison and Kwame Dawes, from whom I learned to see my landscape and society, and to voice in our own rhythms what I observe. As Thompson did, the following locates the Incarnate Christ in my communal life:

The cascading words of my hand
pluck His praise from eight-string bandolin and local banjo,
place His favour on madras and foulard, the satin and the lace,
plant His steps in mazouk, lakonmèt and gwan won;
point His casual grace in yellow pumpkin star, pendular mango,
plait Him a crown of anthurium and fern

And one more:

O – in the beloved corner shrines of mango blossom, breadfruit
palm, almonds' broad oval leaf,
the chapels of sidewalks' hasty awnings, the confessionals of
indignant minivans,
the fuming censer of the streets' sulfur speech –
O, at every wary block – His Real Presence, and archangels
gossiping of His Parousia.
After poems, psalms. And your canticles.

The place of the sacred in poetry is important today since we must be reminded, as Thompson and other writers have shown, of spiritual realities, of the true nature of our fractured planet. As Sherrard puts it, 'An art that possesses a sacred quality is an art that mirrors the miraculous presence of the spiritual world.' And therein is cause for the celebratory, for the hymn, even in our secular, demythologized world.

But Sherrard also points to the serious responsibility of writing the transcendent and immanent and sacred into our poetry and art: 'of this the artist must be sure: that only when his art possesses a sacred quality will it present a positive challenge to our technological world and to the degradation of human life which is endemic to it'.

W S Milne

A Brutal and Primitive Power:
The Poetry of Richard Eberhart

Throughout his writing life Geoffrey Hill paid homage to the poetry of the American Richard Eberhart, rating him highly as a modern poet who fused imaginatively the sensuous world with the metaphysical. As an adolescent Hill would ramble over the Lickey Hills or round by Bewdley and the Severn carrying a copy of Oscar Williams's *A Little Treasury of Modern Poetry* (1946) which included favourite poems by Eberhart and Allen Tate. Whilst at Oxford University, Hill wrote a review of Eberhart's collection, *Undercliff: Poems 1946-1953*, praising the brutal and primitive power of nature evinced in the poetry finely balanced by the structured craft of the verse, qualities evidenced in Hill's own undergraduate poems at the time, some of which were collected in his first book, *For The Unfallen* (1959). From time to time over the years in his essays and lectures Hill would mention the influence of Kierkegaard on his own work, a philosopher-theologian he first read about in Eberhart's poem 'Mysticism Had Not the Patience to Wait for God's Revelation', a quotation from the Danish's writer's extensive canon. Latterly, Geoffrey returned to Eberhart in his Oxford Lectures on Poetry where he again focused on what he called 'the fields of force' (a possible echo of Eberhart's 'Action and Poetry') in this poem, melding, as he thought it did, secular with eternal concerns. For Hill the poem is a meditation on how to escape the subjective lair of the self (the phrase comes from another Eberhart poem) to enter the objective sphere of faith, overcoming 'the heaviness of the world, 'the eternal ape on the leash', causal forces the vatic poet defeats through inspired transcendence. I think it could be argued that Hill's most famous early poem, 'Genesis', owes something to Eberhart's 'The Groundhog', creation in both works evinced as something more than mere pantheism. With these thoughts in mind, let us turn to Eberhart's own writings, exploring some of these themes further.

In his poetry Richard Eberhart (1904–2005) searches for the sacred in the world's corruption, that 'secret hallowing', that 'sudden incarnation', which makes the cosmos (if only for a moment) bearable and understandable. I use the word 'cosmos' advisedly, for the world to Eberhart is more than mere appearance – the spiritual is as real to him as the physical, reaching out to the 'Spiralling wings of Creation', 'the mortal span' as he sees it, in Blakean terms, 'to find out Heaven and Hell'. For him, as for Plato, the temporal world is a perceptible god, beautiful and at times perfect, but also often corrupted, corruptible:

> In June, amid the golden fields,
> I saw a groundhog lying dead...
> Inspecting close his maggots' might
> And seething cauldron of his being,
> Half with loathing, half with a strange love,
> I poked him with an angry stick...
> But the year had lost its meaning,
> And in intellectual chains
> I lost both love and loathing...
> It has been three years, now.
> There is no sign of the groundhog.
> I stood there in the whirling summer,
> My hand capped a withered heart
> And thought of China and Greece,
> Of Alexander in his tent;
> Of Montaigne in his tower,
> Of Saint Theresa in her wild lament.
>   (from 'The Groundhog')

In his essay on Robert Frost he says 'a deep look at appearance will see right through it that there is something behind or beyond the realm of appearance', and in his essay on Theodore Roethke that the poet's task is 'to penetrate the ideal essence behind the mask of time'. At The Fall, man 'uncreated creation', Eberhart writes, by bringing into being the 'putrid lamb' whose 'guts were out for crows to eat', inaugurating our 'crouching hunger' and our 'abysm of suffering'. However, in this post-lapsarian world, transcendence is still possible, for our 'bright mortality' surmounts both the 'Incarcerating sunlight' and the 'churning chaos', bringing 'quick April' and 'whirling summer' with their 'pure mortal breath', the beauty that keeps 'even at the guts of things':

> This fevers me, this sun on green,
> On grass glowing, this young spring.
> The secret hallowing is come,
> Regenerate sudden incarnation,
> Mystery made visible
> In growth yet subtly veiled in all,

Ununderstandable in grass
In flowers, and in the human heart,
This lyric mortal loveliness,
The earth breathing, and the sun.

The poet's duty is 'to shape the intellect/And integrate the spirit',
Eberhart writes, 'to form new shapes' from the Demiurge, and from
'the rich simplicity of the earth' write from 'the full mind stored with
summers', 'speaking the lyric that shall live'. 'The full mind' is not only
that of earthly experience, but an intellectual quality akin to Plato's Eternal
Forms which 'fill' or 'nourish' the soul. 'I dream Plato's dream of being'
he states categorically in one poem, 'human reason directly intuiting the
Divine Reason'. Such 'visionary reason' helps overcome our fear of 'the
terrible void and absolute darkness', 'the axle of the earth', 'the bitten
mind', 'the monstrous passage of the world', 'the separateness of each
man in his lair'. It helps transcend our 'brutal languor' and the 'hours of
leaden torpor'.

The fundamental principle upon which Eberhart's poetry is based is that
of Pascal's insight that 'there are perfections in Nature to show that she
is the image of God and imperfections to show that she is no more than
his image'. So it is the poet obtains rare glimpses into the soul of things,
sudden insights into the essence of the world, free from the bondage
of time and 'the mind's ultimate crevasses' – although this knowledge,
Eberhart acknowledges, can only be confused and partial from our mortal
point of view, in the grip as we are of 'gravid time' and 'the heavy clutch
of memory':

The full day ripens in the sun,
And time has always just begun.
Primeval silence without stir
Holds the earth like gossamer;
For love is slowly blossoming
In quietness too still to sing,
From which all passions green or ripe
Are shadowy blooms of the Immortal Type.
                    (from 'The Bells of a Chinese Temple')

Where are those high and haunting skies,
Higher than the see-through wind? Where are
The rocky springs beyond desire? And where
The sudden source of purity?

Now they are gone again. Though world
Decrease the wraith-like eye so holy,
And bring a summer in, and with it folly,
Though the senses bless and quell,

I would not with such blessings be beguiled,
But seek an image far more dear. Oh where
Has gone that madness wild? Where stays
The abrupt essence and the final shield?

In his prose Eberhart says he is 'religious without belonging to any set church', but that he is 'very sympathetic to all spiritual ideas'. He goes against the modern grain by stating that 'I think that artists should be whole people rather than hurt, broken, mad, or demented ones', but paradoxically believes that 'it's good to be at the pitch that is near madness. That's when you are nearest to the divine insight':

If I could only live at the pitch that is near madness
When everything is as it was in my childhood
Violent, vivid, and of infinite possibility:
That the sun and the moon broke over my head.

Then I cast time out of the trees and fields,
Then I stood immaculate in the Ego;
Then I eyed the world with all delight,
Reality was the perfection of my sight...

To young writers of poetry he says, 'Do not let sociologists, or psychologists, or psychiatrists destroy in us the power to dream. Even daydreaming; that is a part of it'. He adds: 'The deepest things about poetry seem to me to be the mysteries. They go beyond the mind into the vast reservoir and region of the spirit and appear to be not entirely accountable to reason'. His most comprehensive statement of his poetics is to be found in his essay 'Contemporary Authors': 'If we could see or feel beyond the human condition is it possible to think that we could feel or think the unthinkable? The Greeks had aspirations to ideas of immortality. We twentieth century Americans live closer to materialism than to idealism so we are more nearly measurers, like Aristotle, than dreamers of immortal types, like Plato. I am on Plato's side rather than Aristotle's. However, our highest imaginations are ungraspable and we are constantly thrown back into the here and now, into materialistic reality. I think poetry is allied to religion and music. It helps us to live because it expresses our limitations, our mortality, while exciting us to a beyond which may or may not be there'.

'To read the spirit was all my care and is' he writes; 'it is what man does not know of God/Comprises the visible poem of the world':

It was the glimpses in the lightning
Made me a sage, but made me say
No word to make another fight,
My own fighting heart full of dismay.

Spirit, soul, and fire are reached!

... I closed in the wordless ecstasy
Of mystery: where there is no thought
But feeling lost in itself forever,
Profound, remote, immediate, and calm.

So it is the poet, fighting his doubts, seeks 'pure intuition', 'essential unity', 'changeless radiancy', and finds them in poetry's 'final truth' that 'keeps the doors of perception open' to 'the 'hallowed light' of vision, a harmony beyond 'senseless dissonance'. For Eberhart, poetry's making is 'a search for a way to be', helping us to overcome 'the world's heaviness', 'the common land of death'.

The critics have been right to call Eberhart a 'vigorous, idiosyncratic visionary', a poet who seeks 'the impenetrable text of reality', 'a stubborn individualist who also is one of the most authentically gifted and instinctively poetic minds of our time'. His is a poetry we must continue to read and enjoy, not least for its profound apprehensions of the sacred, for its breaking of our 'strong, dread solitude', 'the long suffering that knows no close':

But in the great moments of being, something
Beyond our wills, is the prime mover
And we do not deny this when we bring
Passionate love to a woman, as a lover...

In its temporality ('the grandeur of the actual') the poetry of Richard Eberhart paradoxically discovers a vision of the eternal beyond this 'world of broken strangeness'.

Tony Roberts

Al Alvarez at Risk

'If you ask me what I came to do in this world, I, an artist, will answer you:
"I am here to live out loud."'
(Zola)

Al Alvarez is in high profile once again, as others evaluate his contribution
to poetry criticism from the late nineteen fifties on. In a long life he has been
highly influential, but particularly for his stint as the poetry editor and critic
for *The Observer* and through his anthology *The New Poetry* (1962), the
Penguin Modern European Poets series (from 1967) and *The Savage God:
A Study in Suicide* (1971). Essentially Alvarez promoted American poets
like Robert Lowell, John Berryman and then, perhaps most importantly,
Sylvia Plath. He also introduced many British readers to what were called
– in Churchill's popular metaphor – 'Iron Curtain' poets. Despite other
contending perspectives, Alvarez's own tastes were dominant. He offered a
view of poetry as disciplined, exciting and risky – and risk was very much
to the taste of the time.

It is hardly surprising then that he should title his selected essays in 2007
Risky Business – albeit that the title firstly addresses the perils of freelancing
– since risk has been a great stimulus to his own writing and reading, as well
as to his other pursuits. Influenced by Freud's contentions about conflict in
the psyche, Alvarez has been remarkably consistent in the view that 'Risk
concentrates the mind, sharpens the senses and, in every way, makes life
sweeter by putting it, however briefly, in doubt.' To him, 'risk' in poetry
is a central feature of Modernism. It is about letting air into what he refers
ironically to as 'the hallowed tradition'. In an essay on Derek Walcott for
the the *New York Review of Books*, in 2000, Alvarez referred to the Nobel
Prize winner as being in the Victorian tradition: 'He is not an experimental
poet and has never been easy with the fast-talking, hard-edged high anxiety
that gives the Modernist writers their peculiar sense of strain.' Again, in *The
Writer's Voice* (2005), he defined Extremism (aka risk) as 'an art that goes
out along that friable edge between the tolerable and intolerable, yet does so
with all the discipline and clarity and attention to detail Eliot implied when
he talked of Classicism'.

The roots of risk were in Alvarez's personality and personal circumstances.
In a 1992 essay titled he wrote: 'In my early thirties, after my first marriage
broke up, I acquired a brief reputation as a wild man: I drove fast cars,

played high stakes poker, and spent more time than I decently could afford off in the hills, climbing rocks with the boys.' The obverse of this is his sense of the staid. It is reflected in Alvarez's disenchantment with English as a student at Oxford, where he found the lit. crit. old-fashioned (unlike Cambridge where F. R. Leavis, I. A. Richards and William Empson were active in the same way as the New Critics in America, influenced by Richards and T. S. Eliot in liberating the text from its author's ownership).

With honourable exceptions (such as D. H. Lawrence) British poetry had shied away from Modernism, Alvarez began to feel, and with it recognition of vital twentieth century preoccupations (the influence of Freud, the concentration camps, Existentialism). In *The Shaping Spirit* (1958) he wrote 'in the very broadest terms... modernism has been predominantly an American concern, a matter of creating, almost from scratch, their own poetic tradition. It has affected English poetry peculiarly little.' His 1980 piece on Seamus Heaney in the *New York Review of Books* ('beautiful minor poetry') echoed the same disenchantment:

Apart from Joyce and Becket, the great experimental movement in literature was largely an American concern. In contrast, the British adjusted to the times by a process of seepage, gradually adapting the old forms to the rhythms of twentieth century speech: Yeats, Auden, Graves, and so on, down to Larkin. So they are comfortable with Heaney because he himself is comfortably in a recognizable tradition.

In an essay on T.E. Hulme and Wilfred Owen in the same magazine he suggests that the fact that a generation had been slaughtered in the trenches might have a bearing on this, adding that 'The line of English verse in the 20th century runs directly from the Victorians, via Hardy and Housman, to Larkin and Hughes, almost as if Modernism had never happened.'

With a sense that contemporary British poetry and criticism having failed him, Alvarez turned to America as early as 1953. 'It was love at first sight', he wrote in his autobiography, *Where Did It All Go Right?* (1999): 'I loved the energy of the place, the busyness and cynicism of New York and the intellectual openness, even in staid Princeton' (where he experienced what the theoretical physicist Freeman Dyson had described as a post-war world for the young 'without shadows'). There he was to deliver the Christian Gauss lectures at the age of twenty-eight. He also fell under the spell of Richard Blackmur, 'one of the first and most original of the New Critics', Kenneth Burke and others. Later he was also to establish a friendship with Robert Lowell.

Alvarez's highly influential *Observer* years had begun in 1956. The reviews helped establish him and, beginning in 1959 with R.S. Thomas, the paper also began publishing poems by well-established poets, and then

Hughes, Gunn and Americans like Lowell, Berryman and Roethke. What he did not want, he made clear in one of his *Observer* columns:

The style of the fifties is now achieved and accepted: that is, a large number of poets write in much the same way and share much the same emotional stance: a no-nonsense, let's-get-down-to-it, common-chappery, determinedly competent and determinedly restrained. Where Modernist posts used to rally to Ezra Pound's war cry, "Poetry should be at least as well written as prose," they now settle for more Somerset Maughamish principles, as who should say, "A poem should have a beginning, a middle and an end."' (June 19, 1960)

As William Wootten notes, in *The Alvarez Generation: Thom Gunn, Geoffrey Hill, Ted Hughes, Sylvia Plath and Peter Porter* (2015), Alvarez became the critic 'as commentator, populariser or provocateur'. His anthology, *The New Poetry*, helped secure the British reputations of two (and, in the revised edition of 1968, four) American poets, while many contemporary British poets, like those involved in The Movement, were in effect damned with faint praise.

What lit the fuse of *The New Poetry* was Alvarez's introductory essay (with its Freudian homage) 'Beyond the Gentility Principle'. As he explained in *Risky Business*, 'I wrote it in 1961, a particularly dreary moment in British poetry, in the hope of stirring things up.' Our poets, he felt, offered 'a tetchy vision of post-war provincial England populated, like a Lowry painting, by stick figures united, above all, by boredom.' The essay calls for an Arnoldian 'new seriousness' to take modern poetry forward: 'I would define this seriousness simply as the poet's ability and willingness to face the full range of his experience with his full intelligence'. (The argument was influenced, according to Wootten, by Harold Rosenberg's seminal comments on American painting and culture in *The Tradition of the New, 1959.*) Alvarez recognised a negativity in the 50s 'Movement': 'academic-administrative verse, polite, knowledgeable, efficient, polished, and, in its quiet way, even intelligent.' Bloodless, in other words. Circumstances might change, he believed, the class system might disturb the surface calm, but Britain remained impervious to events and ideas. In short, 'the concept of gentility still reigns supreme'. Gentility, as he later explained, 'didn't seem an adequate response to a century that had spawned two world wars, totalitarianism, genocide, concentration camps and nuclear warfare'.

'The Movement' poets had been so dubbed by *The Spectator* in 1954 and initially including Kingsley Amis, Donald Davie, Philip Larkin, Elizabeth

Jennings, John Wain and Robert Conquest. Although he featured some of them in *The New Poetry*, to Alvarez 'The Movement' poets represented all that was unadventurous and xenophobic about contemporary British verse:

For Amis & Co., Modernism was a plot by foreigners – Americans, Irishmen and Continentals, people with funny accents they could mimic – to divert literature from its true purpose; and their business was to get it back on its traditional track, back to Arnold Bennett and Galsworthy, back to Chesterton, Hardy and Housman. (*Where Did It All Go Right?*)

The two best Movement-associated poets were, for him, Philip Larkin and Thom Gunn. Wootten quotes Alvarez's comment on Larkin's under-achievement in not having 'mapped out any great new continent of poetry' but 'simply to have created a tone of voice for the time'. This was a judgment from 1958 and again it is a shying away from the demands of literary Modernism, of risk, that is at stake. This was the case also in *The New Poetry* essay, where Hughes's energy ('a nexus of fear and sensation') was favoured over Larkin's accomplished restraint. Although Alvarez recognised Larkin's eminence among his British peers, it was coupled with the feeling that the poet had 'a beady understanding' of his own limitations. The fact that he had not been represented by more poems in *The New Poetry* was to do with permission fees, however, not craft.

Alvarez had admired Thom Gunn's early poetry for its technical control and subject matter. In exploring 'psychic pain' Gunn belonged with Alvarez's risk takers, but when the poet moved to California and came under the influence of Ivor Winters, whose antipathy to the New Critics was well-known, Alvarez began to feel that 'The unease and energy that had made the early poems tick so ominously gave way to decorum, strict reasonableness and formal grace – to smoothly flowing rhythms and bland rhymes.' Gunn's technique was finally redeemed, for the critic, by the fine elegies in his last book, *The Man With Night Sweats* (1992), written to friends who died of AIDS.

Although some of Alvarez's judgments seem harsh, unfair, there were those who agreed with him about 'The Movement'. As David Perkins wrote in *A History of Modern Poetry* (1987): 'Even poets who had been featured in the Movement anthologies were snipping at the "tame," "academic," "arid," "mean spirited" style and ethos the anthologies had promoted.' Perkins sees poets such as David Jones, Bail Bunting and Charles Tomlinson as otherwise being outside their 1950s orthodoxy.

Now Alvarez turned in his introductory essay in *The New Poetry* to the example of American poets Robert Lowell and John Berryman who, while learning from Eliot, nevertheless rejected his idea of 'impersonality', turning the focus frankly on themselves. So, he later recounted, 'I put the two

Americans at the beginning [of the anthology] in order to set a standard, as an antidote to the complacency of the Movement, as a deliberate provocation.'

Alvarez had taken to Robert Lowell's work early, seeing the 'dis-ease' beneath its carapace of Catholic symbolism. In *The Shaping Spirit* (1958) he wrote of Lowell and Lowell's one-time teacher, Richard Eberhart: 'Both Eberhart and Lowell have worked with considerable power to make of their obscure emotional disturbances a matter of more general and deliberate truth.' When Lowell's brilliant *Life Studies* (1959) appeared in England, Alvarez recognised its worth immediately. As he remembers in his autobiography: 'Instead of rounding up the usual suspects in 800 words, I wrote a much longer article on Lowell's book alone.' Alvarez would maintain his commitment to Lowell's verse for its technical accomplishments as well as for its courage *in extremis*. He felt that the 'inwardness' of poets like him (and later Plath) when confronting their demons was not a turning from the world but a way of reflecting the 'bewildering nihilism' consequent upon the Second World War. In *The Savage God* Alvarez even compared *Life Studies* to *The Waste Land* for its courage and revolutionary innovation. Behind it was his frustration at British criticism of the time, as well as the poetry. He wrote in 1977 of having been irked that 'In Britain [Lowell's] originality was acknowledged, but grudgingly, as though it were not quite the done thing for a serious poet to lay himself on the line so nakedly.'

Alvarez also praised John Berryman's best poetry very highly, again for the inventive risks it took in exploring its author's angst. Berryman speaks through his alcoholic, picaresque hero, Henry, a man with 'badly frayed nerves and an unremitting case of morning-after guilt'. Berryman's suicide in 1972 (after Plath's of nine years before) gave Alvarez pause for thought. In the *New York Times* he wrote:

> For years I have been extolling the virtues of what I have called extremist poetry, in which artists deliberately push their perceptions to the very edge of the tolerable. Both Berryman and Sylvia Plath were masters of the style. But knowing now how they both died I no longer believe that any art – even that as fine as they produced at their best – is worth the terrible cost.

Yet Alvarez's partiality for risk had influenced him against other poets, whatever their status (as we saw with Heaney). For instance, he concluded a less than impressed *Observer* review of Wallace Stevens in February 1960 with the words: 'The idea that art could come from immersing in the destructive element never seems to have occurred to him. It is as though he had never really *read* Shakespeare.'

Eventually Alvarez turned from his favoured American 'extremist' poets to what he considered the even higher seriousness of Central European practice. During his time at *The Observer*, he would feature groups of poems in translation. Through his connection to the BBC Third Programme he journeyed to Warsaw to write a feature on intellectual life and met Zbigniew Herbert, who became a good friend. He followed up with features on Czechoslovakia, Hungary and Yugoslavia. This led in turn to Penguin initiating the 'Penguin Modern European Poets' series, with which Alvarez was connected for 12 years and 22 volumes. He wrote introductions for two of the collections, those by Miroslav Holub (1967) and Herbert (1968). Given the political conditions in Czechoslovakia and Poland at the time, risk was the métier of these poets. Alvarez wrote of the first:

In its way, Holub's poetry is no less exploratory than that of the Extremist poets of the West, but it takes the opposite direction. His business is with the way in which private responses, private anxieties, connect up with the public world of science, technology and machines.

In a recent 'Commentary' essay for the *The Times Literary Supplement*, Justin Quinn has criticised Alvarez's failure to recognise in Holub's poetry the influence of the Beats, despite Holub's insistence on that influence. The significance of the criticism is for Quinn that Alvarez 'rescues a public voice for poetry, but only writers from communist regimes are allowed to write it'.

Alvarez had the highest opinion of Zbigniew Herbert's poetry, reckoning in 1985 that it was better, even in translation, than that of anyone writing in England or America. He was deeply influenced by Herbert's classicism and dangerous anti-establishment perspective: 'He had been inventing and overthrowing gods ever since, as a party of one, he was permanently and warily in opposition.' For Alvarez, Herbert had 'a moral authority which poets in the West lacked'. In fact it had made him feel 'shabby' and 'pompous' for ever having called for a 'new seriousness' when he read Herbert. 'Now I was faced with a poet with a different scale of values,' he wrote. Whether or not the needs of post-war poetry were the same in Poland and England, as Wootten queries, it does not alter the fact that Alvarez brought these poets to a large audience in Britain. He also wrote persuasively on other European poets in translation, like Vladimir Mayakovsky ('a genius for exhibitionism') and Czesław Miłosz (suffering 'the vacuum of exile').

Arguably, the two poets who gained most from Alvarez's support – and most controversially – were Sylvia Plath and Ted Hughes. According to his account in *Where Did It All Go Right?* after ten years he had had a 'bellyful of poets' and turned to other books, novels and magazine pieces, but first came *The Savage God: A Study of Suicide* which contributed to the legend around Sylvia Plath.

Alvarez had met Plath through her husband, Ted Hughes, though he was initially more impressed with the excellent early poetry of Hughes. In *The Savage God* he wrote of these poems, 'They seemed to emerge from an absorbed, physical world that was wholly his own.' With his first two books, *The Hawk in the Rain* and *Lupercal*, 'A figure had emerged on the drab scene of British poetry, powerful and undeniable'. Alvarez was aware of the connection in Hughes between 'the violence both of animal life and of the self... It was almost as though, despite all the reading and polish and craftsmanship, he had never properly been civilized'.

Gradually, as the friendships developed, Alvarez came to recognise and respect Sylvia Plath's poetry. In *The Savage God* he recounts how he warmed to *The Colossus*, to 'the precision and concentration with which she handled language, the unemphatic range of vocabulary, her ear for subtle rhythms, and her... rhymes'. Once a student of Lowell's and now married to Hughes, the couple were 'intent on finding voices for their unquiet, buried selves'. In an article on Ted Hughes's *Birthday Letters* in 1998, Alvarez explained how 'Hughes calls her father "The Minotaur" and a large number of the *Birthday Letters* chart Plath's gradual, fatal descent into his lair.' As he describes it, it was Hughes who showed her how to get there and he did it in the name of poetry.

Plath of course transcended her influences. She was a brilliant, original poet who wrote poems with courage and insight that were 'proved on her pulses'. Hughes and Alvarez were there at a crucial period. They contributed to her reputation by their encouragement and promotion.

Although Alvarez did not know this at the time, Plath was in the last days of her life when she came to him for help as friend and editor. As a guest on radio's 'Desert Island Discs', he put his inability to recognise her clinical depression down as 'stupidity' and, characteristically, added:

And the more subtle reason is that her poems were so good and there was such liveliness. I mean, there was more life and liveliness and appetite in Plath writing about death than there is in the collected works of Philip Larkin writing about what a bitch it is to be alive.

Subsequently, *The Savage God* offers a long, involving and disturbing late portrait of Plath. It is a portrayal which did not go unchallenged. Ted Hughes wrote to Alvarez, in November 1971, deploring the appearance of extracts from it in *The Observer,* and with some justification, because of the revelation of intimate details of Plath's suicide. He blamed Alvarez for turning the children's 'guardian angel' into a 'public statue' for others to gawk at. Alvarez could only point out, as he did, that it had been 'written with great care and as a tribute to Sylvia'. In fact he had gone as far as to compare her prolific last months to Keats' 'marvellous year'. He had neither sensationalised nor criticised, but the account was inevitably intrusive.

Alvarez has had several opportunities to express his insights into Plath's work and personality. In his autobiography, for example, he returned to the irony he noted in his radio interview: 'But the poems she wrote in her suicidal depression are sardonic, angry, unforgiving, tender, yet disciplined and always curiously detached; they are full of life, not death.' Above all Alvarez has remained alert to the injustice to Plath that a misreading of her life has meant to her and her poetry. In the pages of the *New York Review of Books* in 1989 he deplored Anne Stevenson's biography *Bitter Fame* for turning Plath into a suicidal 'monster'. He rejected the 'cult' of Plath as being 'based on the suicide rather than on the pure, disciplined, hard-edged poems' and was disgusted at her misuse as a feminist cause, which he felt involved 'the crudest sentimentality'.

Al Alvarez has always been a controversial figure, which he doubtless relishes. His critics challenge the idea that poetry needs to be wedded to anxiety, risk and extremism. With the passage of time other anthologies have had their say (including Bloodaxe's 2002 bestseller, the appropriately titled *Staying Alive*). Also, Alvarez's favourite poets are increasingly becoming their biographies, especially given the near-inseparability of their lives and work. And, most obviously, other poets are in the spotlight: John Ashbery, Seamus Heaney and Paul Muldoon among them. Philip Larkin, Ted Hughes and, most recently, Geoffrey Hill have been canonised, and Britain's most popular living poets – Carol Ann Duffy and Simon Armitage – hold centre stage.

If poetry lives the second time as biography, this is true too for a handful of critics, also. Today we are as apt to read *about* T.S. Eliot, F. R. Leavis, William Empson, Lionel Trilling and Edmund Wilson as read their work. Harold Bloom will soon face similar treatment. Al Alvarez too is beginning to draw attention for his active participation in the events of the time. After all, Wootten's book is not named *The Alvarez Generation* for nothing. Justin Quinn, reviewing it in the *Times Literary Supplement*, observed, 'Like his favoured and favourite poets, Alvarez has had the gift of making his own preoccupations those of the age.' But to give the last quote to the infinitely quotable man himself (who until very recently swam in the ponds of Hampstead Heath each morning): 'Freud has written, "Life loses in interest, when the highest stake in the game of living, life itself, may not be risked."'

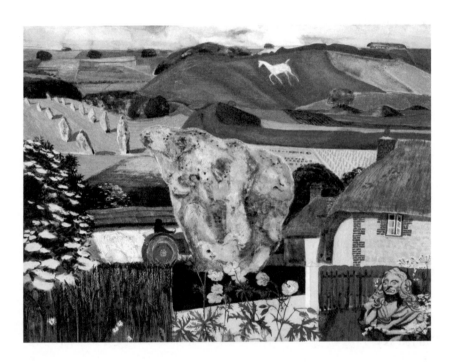

William Bedford

The Flitting

i.m. John Clare

Skaiting

There was a field where frost's come,
cobwebs white, grass white,
ground gone,
overnight,

new mirror for dazzling sun.
Now skaiters waltz – laugh – cry –
skreek like magpie
passing by.

I skait across my mind,
tek falls no skaiter understands,
read winter words
in red sky.

Sit on farm gate
that fences heaven round,
no trespasses allowed for larks
or rabbit pie.

There was a field where frost's come,
new owner of the heath,
pasture ground,
rainbows in the free sky.

skaiting skating *skreek* shriek, scream

Wopstraw Clack

He liked Mary, folks say. Talked to her.
Gawped in Seaton's classroom.
Lost work dreaming tales better not dreamt.

Liked trees too, willows 'specially,
the way they leaned out over water,
reaching for t'other side. Daft, some folk said.

He allus liked Mary.
Followed her home, though her wouldn't listen.
His youthful crush, blushy youngen.

Her fether knew better.
Martha was the one he married.
Called her Patty. His good woman.

He hadn't heard Mary died.
Went walking home, flitting asylum.
His other wife on his mind. Woody nightshade.

wopstraw country bumpkin *clack* chatter, gossip *Mary* Mary Joyce, his
childhood sweetheart *Martha* Martha Turner, Clare's wife, known by him
as Patty.

We Never Met

John Clare to John Keats

We never met,
missed by chance,
though you more comfortable
where poets meet than me,
farmyards and fields my close familiars.

Then death looked by,
you at sea, me back at home.
Taylor said you wrote:
my Images from Nature
not called by any living Sentiment.

Best criticism I ever received,
words not to be thrown away.
I read your Chaucer, Taylor's own copy.
So poets to poets,
across a much wider sea.

Take Your Own Trundle

Crows bate me,
scarecrow boy unbrunt
by glabbering lords,
ladies' whews,

I shut my mind to crows
preachin' pews
noise
the clatterin' hawks chasin' food.

Mary's watchet eyes
watch me with sad surprise,
old cart carting love
to paradise.

take your own trundle go your own way *bate* harass *unbrunt* unhindered
by glabbering chattering *whews* the cry of birds, or imitating the cry of
birds *watchet* light blue

Vuyelwa Carlin

Scarista Beach, Isle of Harris

for Netty

The wind, so powerful
– your last year, who could know? – the sea
writhed, white and grey: waul of milling,

bobbing birds. We leaned back on sprung air,
trusting the wind. Salty, soaked, you roamed and roamed,
glutted with seascape – wouldn't leave

that huge roaring beach, the sand
blown hard as flint. How aching-cold the hissing water –
out there, little icy slippy heads

of fascinated seals. – Scarista House requests, politely,
no TV on the Sabbath; long, bluey
windy dusks of treeless Harris, core of blue-lit

midnight sky. Pellucid Gaelic vowels
sang from the kitchen. – Later, another midnight,
you died, stiff with frost, the nearby Onny

tinkling with flimsy ice. – Brittle in earth;
a silver cross, a picture of your boy: I have that night's clothes
– the coat's torn lining – drift of White Musk –

rolled up behind your notebooks,
photos, reading glasses (those odd, bright-red rims).
You had humility; hosts of friends: Psalm 131,

stuck on your mirror: *Lord,
my heart is not haughty, nor mine eyes lofty*: –
rigorous Harris, its wind-plucked boulder-fields, the ringing sand.

Sharon Black

West Highland

If I were to lie back, this is the landscape I'd become –
blanched tussocks, copses of pine,
shining lochs, station platform signs translated
to a language I can't pronounce;

lazy fences, serious houses, two shaggy rams
grazing by a pleated auburn stream,
alder, beech and dithery aspen,
Munros shouldering the last lost weight of snow;

a blaze of gorse along the verge, pylons marching
over bog and moor, the ninety-six miles we walked last year
with backache, slippery from sweat and midge spray,
the craic of good friends keeping us upright

as we lost and found the Way.

Anne Ryland

The Singing Women of Duddo

Their welcome was stark. 'Northumberland's hinny',
as I announced myself, left them unconvinced.
With my basket of frets I hunkered beside the sockets
of the missing two, who also managed to impart aloofness.
The five survivors were staring outwards at the restive Cheviots

loss running down their faces, their expressions still in use
when no one else was up on this wind-shorn hill.
September the first; these women were waiting for winter,
winter that had tapered them, written them – circles of praises,
linear criticisms. Their huddle hinted at secrets.

Too far off an unmarked path, though, to be my sisters.
A reading class perhaps, of slow-rolling hill-stories
or a splinter group sworn to listening; no wittering.
An assembly of the menless, the bairnless, the in-mourning?
Wind-stripped now, I had to address the mardy sandstone ladies

in my East Saxon voice, from Beamfleote – confessed
I was an exile in this land of hats and boots, its dialect
dusted with slack, and I was seeking Neolithic counsel.
Their silence, somewhere between a rejection and a sanctuary,
whittled me down to my quietest quiet, and urged me to go.

I hadn't heard the women earn their other name
by singing four-thousand-year-old Northumbrian notes,
their own low, whistling so-so-so-ing when the wind
vibrated through their fluted bodies; gingerly I descended
to Duddo, imagining that song unfurling mine.

My daughter no longer needed me to read her stories

after a paper sculpture by Su Blackwell

Each evening I'd watch her climb her little ladder of words
then a *Ha,* an *Ooh* or spatter of laughter.

The more she read and read, her book-bed rose and rose.
Down at floorboard level, I almost heard her eyes sweeping
castles, forests, islands, and myself squealing.
The pink room I'd grown for her turned feverish.

I caught her struggling to scale the tall shadow-ladder.
Her enchantment repainted the ceiling magenta
and I could only study it, a bloodshot winter sunset.
But the girl balanced on her library, too far to decipher.

What if the books collapsed in a heap of unhappy endings?
How had she conquered that stockpile of volumes?
She was sleeping, living, on peculiar novels
foreign to me. I suspected my daughter dreamed
in chapters, leaping from one to the next in a paper-coat.

Tempting to remind her who had taught her.
Instead I told myself: all stories are damp with departures.
Back to her wall, I composed postcards
to her in the dark. Any night now she'd fly out
on the breath of her mothy wings.

Paul Murray

The Spirit Eel

The baby died. A vein burst in his head.
A spirit eel wriggled free from the cupped minds
Of his carers, downstream to the Dead:
A ribbon unravelling in the tie that binds...

We are all liquid in life, liquidly held,
In the balance, liquidly we slip the leash,
Pendulous raindrops whose sides have swelled
About to set a trick of light to crash.

Drawn to our communal coma, past all heed,
A spawn of sleep from which there is no waking,
Sperm and egg swim against Time's tide to breed,
We trickle through fingers of our own making.

Rosalind Hudis

What the Burglar Took

That night it was nothing.
Cinematic, he'd slid
under the kitchen window,
swerved an old veined saucer,
rocked the vintage cactus,
slippered his way across tiles
on a moulting rug
that still smelt of your last dog
and made you wheeze.

After that threshold no sign,
yet you felt him in every omission -
the carriage clock that paced him
but never chimed, silver fish
partying by moonlight who'd fled
into covens of dust, slivers
of street-lamp that laid a grid
from back to front room
where shadows failed to creak.

His exit, another window,
half open in the study.
The room was rigid with night,
The Great Bear
encrypted in the cushions.
You touched frost on the inside,
took to spying on your house,
heard whispers in the heating kettle
morse in the water-pipes.

Nick Burbridge

Matriarch

The undertaker poses gamely while her posse
bear the wicker basket to the run then takes the stand
to simper through her homily chock-full of cliché
and botched fact, capped with a homespun ditty
to mothers the world over: witless pantomime.

The family pitch in with poems and songs.
Only the cracked son in his back pew
rubs his hands fiercely between his thighs
and cries, *What is this?* –
swiftly silenced by his wife's dry palm.

It is the hour when issues close, the shelter
of the crematorium. But in his depths
huge sluice gates open, currents flail,
loosing the quick tow and tide
the dead one always stirred in him,
so to escape the swell that dragged him down,
by old age, he had learned to fix her,
in his mind's eye, as a roped mule
stranded in a quarry far inland
he visited on feast days only,
looking down the steep stone wall
where she turned weary circles
grinding her loneliness, thirsting for his touch,
though he stayed out of reach, since, for him
even the rush of her tears was too much.

Now he prays last hours of contrition
when it seemed she had shrivelled
to a safe point will redeem him.
None could prise him from her shoulder then;
he stroked her white hair, cradling her head;
and when oblivion pressed down on her
whispered stories in her whorled ear
told him long before, where errant whales,

guided by pure sound,
crossed vast oceans
to recover their lost schools,
mimicking her tone,
so the last strains she heard
were hushed parables they shared alone,
whether she welcomed it or not.

It seemed to work. When he was left
with her beached corpse he saw her
transfigured in the lamplight,
found, perfected, or resolved.
He wondered that he'd somehow given birth,
kept murmuring, Well done, well done,
as if she'd passed an acid test,
sang fragments of *O Come, O Come Emmanuel,*
Close The Door, They're Coming In the Window –
until nurses moved in to transport her,
his eyes fixed on the gold ring curled
on her cold finger, he recalled another fable
of the seas, claimed it for himself
and, pressing it into his palm,
he bent and asked, *Is this enough?*

Now, as curtains twitch and furnace roars,
he turns the plaited metal through
his own chilled fingers in his pocket
like a rosary that keeps him locked in prayer.

Yet when rollers creak and coffin rocks
he slumps, as if he has been shot,
struck in discombobulating waves
by the full weight and depth of her,
the sheer scope of all her years
meeting claim and need so fluently
she surged into the lives of others
on a tide that pulls and drives them still;
while he appears as a mere mote in the lining
of her purse, lodged too tight to separate,
too easily detached to be devout.

This is the cracked man's curse:
not that his delusions lack love's thrust,
or the heaving that he triggers may be false.
But waves round him swell and beat
with such force they can't be held;
the urge to bear him in time banished
by the need for him to be cut out.

So from the closed ranks of mourners
as he's pulled towards the light of day
and the relief of oxygen, he shies,
and dare not tell himself the new voice
he hears among the tumult in his head
is hers, more dominant yet pained than ever;
for it bears her answer in a sentence with no end:
too little, son, too late, too little, son...

Arcadian

To turn back shows no lack of due respect
for the order of the living or the dead.
This border is not mounted to deflect
what should be reasoned, or what must be said.
It's just that I am weary of the cost.

It may be your thrust that passing years'
endeavour, juggling with our joy or grief
should wisen us; or constant trials and fears
confer some status. It's not my belief.
I think old age falls round us like a frost.

No concept lifts us with the subtle urge
of innocence regained, or tenderness
recovered through impulse and need that surge
through us, if we keep faith in nakedness.
I sense we are best found when we are lost.

It's no triumph to have ideas to burn,
causes to follow, strategies to prove
or journeys to achieve, if we don't learn
what we pursue we pass with every move.
It was in simple acts we learned to trust.

It's not too late to return; this is no land
to stake out, but a state forgotten; clasp
me gently, in old ways; we'll understand
full well what we are; it's in our grasp.
I vow we will not leave until we're lost.

John Mole

Across the World

How vulnerable our little gatherings
to a change in the weather, how suddenly
wind and rain gather their strength outside
and then become an inner howl
that breaks the glass. A full moon's face
is at the window, its drenched reflection
inconsolable, not begging to come in
but here already as of right, as pale as death
from across the world, to warm itself
beside a fire too lovingly built up
where ash and flickering residual flames
lay waste the crumbs of comfort.

However we arrange our china plates
they cannot hide a fault line
opening across the table, however
we spread the cloth a tremor
lifts it. Our fragile, ritual domesticities
will not protect us from the towering
wave of conscience or the tide
that swells as it recedes and carries
everything we thought was ours alone
towards oblivion. So happiness is luck,
and loss no less the possibility
that what may never happen surely does.

The Counterpoint

Momentum, melody, miraculous surprise
of wordless utterance rings out
the beautiful changes as we sound them
reaching for analogies. How each note
marked by time and keeping it becomes
a pilgrim shaking off the burden
of unanswered prayer. Or suddenly,
its deep breath liberally exhaled,
draws music from the well where echoes
gather in anticipation, joining
to begin a song, familiar though
never before so clear, the counterpoint
of loss accepted and the gift of grace.

Jill Townsend

Water Torture

Light rain pricks the sea mass
as if it were a doll to be tormented
and, as if expressing pain,
the points radiate out
becoming circles, dissipate
as best they can the suffering.

What distresses the sky so
to generate the crying?
Is there some consolation in this
pricking and nipping at another's skin;
does it reach out to the true
tormentor wherever, whoever it is?

Surfacing

She came up through bubbles of days,
each shiny and unique with experience;
it was as if you could hold them
in your hand, turn them, be dazzled.
Many had a dark twist in the middle
like the glass marbles we played with as children.
But they all hurried past together, bubbles
releasing the air, the days, from her lungs.
Other bubbles merged, from other swimmers:
it was a blizzard in a glass dome.
Only when something took it up and shook it
did she start to feel alone.

David Cooke

Ode to Cobalt

The fact you are named
for a demon enhances
your mystique.

The most sublime
of metals and source
of deepest
blue, you were
unearthed
in disappointment
by men intent
on silver.

In ores mixed
with arsenic,
you bided your time,
releasing
noxious fumes.
Unyielding,
you disdain
those whose sight
is bleared.

To the earthbound,
the visionless,
you gave no hint
of who you were
or any link
to Pharaoh's tomb
where coloured glass
opened up
cerulean vistas.

Before we tagged
or categorized you
your glazes
altered
common clay
into the vases,
plates

and dishes
of Chinese
imperial palaces.

Self-willed, ambivalent,
you bared your soul
reluctantly
to those who'd learn
your secrets
and once dissolved
in glycerol
your writing
can't be read
until the page
is warmed.

Most of the time
you're harmless;
but now
we've glimpsed
your reckless side
you could be
our downfall,
reducing all we are
to dust.

In fish, eggs and liver
your presence
sustains us.
Without you
we're nothing –
if our blood
should thin
and our nerves
falter.

Feeding the brain,
you've shaken up
our least
inspired thinking.

Untramelled,
serene,
you are like
the truth,
that frees us.

Christopher Meredith

In this stilled air the turning trees

In this stilled air
   the turning trees
      it seems are waiting.

Even the birch that flickered tinsel
even the nervy feathers of ash
   hang still
      and all the woodland has become
the picture of its own slow patience.

Not that the music's stopped.
In sap that's slowing
      under bark
obedient to the
      tilt of earth
in leaves that microfractionally curl
the tiny modulations
   still must work

      but the orchestra's so close to mute
the submerged beat so slowed
it takes you to the edge of sense
where sound and memory and self dispute
             identities
      before some new crescendo to
a haemorrhage can come

and you know your own blood's whisper
 – *lob* it says, and *dub* it says –
      is the whisper of the world

   and still it stands
   and still, as Galileo almost said, it moves
 this music of the shape we make in time
the almost
      stillness of the air
we have to play.

Tim Murdoch

Villanelle

Only the light, pure empathy, abides;
not fire, nor filament, nor frosted glass.
Reflection flatters to deceive; divides.

One half on show, the other half it hides,
a moon pretends to burn like molten brass.
Only the light, pure empathy, abides.

Your kind face unintentionally derides
images that look way above my class.
Reflection flatters to deceive; divides.

Careless, nature by miracle provides
star debris, sunspots, seasonal as grass.
Only the light, pure empathy, abides.

Theosophists, seekers with spirit guides,
quest for a vision that has come to pass.
Reflection flatters to deceive; divides.

Sailors, surfers, foresee the dangerous tides.
Intention, back in time, turns into farce.
Only the light, pure empathy, abides.
Reflection flatters to deceive; divides.

Gill Learner

Heiligenstadt and After

I would have put an end to my life –
only art it was that withheld me.
                    Ludwig van Beethoven

Day and night starlings roosted in his skull, bees
infested his brain; a violin's high Es were lost.
Friends mumbled: he withdrew from company.
Once, he could have heard a leaf drop onto grass,
now the world was fading. He tried almond oil, herbs,
blistering of the arms; left the clatter of *fiaker*-wheels
for village life, was always alert for news of cures.

But what he'd prized above all else was lost:
how could he play a keyboard that didn't sing; how
conduct an orchestra that mimed? Although notes
filled his head, cascaded onto staves in symphonies,
concertos, string quartets, still the eternal question:
Müss es sein? And the unforgiving answer:
                    Es müss sein.

The Genius from Pisa

The scented smoke is dizzying, even in Duomo cool.
Padre Benito drones: *Dominus vobiscum.* A young man
drags his thoughts from the purple flowerings
on the cleric's face – syphilis, for sure – responds
Et cum spirito tuo. Dare he, a mere student, advise
a dose of mercury? He yawns, shakes his head,
notices two altar lamps swaying in a draught.
The smaller swings higher and yet they are in time.
He presses fingers to his wrist, checks them against
his pulse, sits up with a jerk: what if there were
a clock that worked by pendulum...

At seventy-eight, forbidden by the Church
to leave his home, he sits in a patch of sun, relives
some high-lights of his life: works on harmonic oscillation;
improvements to the telescope; behaviour of the moons
of Jupiter, and his heresy – confirmation that the earth
moves round the sun. He remembers the Duomo lamps,
gropes for a pen, sighs. His son, Vincenzio soothes:
I'll be your eyes: tell me what to draw. The old man
describes a cog-wheel and two curving pawls which will be
flicked up by a pendulum and also keep it on the move –
the workings of his clock.

Peter Dale

Smithereens

Nocturnal memories of where I never was,
a stranger telling me I know not what,
     the glinting smithereens of the years past,
     then such kaleidoscopes, now fallen apart,
broken beer-bottles, medicine- and wine-
Metaphors, no clue to where, who or why.
     Disjunctive jigsaw bits that won't extrapolate
     to give full pictures of message, person, place.

Optical illusions of the mind's eye
or peripheral glimpses, preconscious sights,
     eye-corners, from the missing bygone scenes
     that mind can't coax the memory to see.
Place, persons, times grow more and more opaque.
Hindsight can't put the scrambled tesserae straight.

William Oxley

On a Blackbird Nesting in my Garden

Flittering to and from your nest in hedge
Oblivious of cat or human near,
I am reminded once more of making's mystery
By your self-effacing simple care
And persistent gathering of material everywhere:
A writhing worm within your beak's sharp wedge
Or insect snapped to its last brief misery,
Or wisp of dead grass borne through air
To mend maybe some wind-forced split
In your secret branch-supported basket.

In deep concentration of being in sun or rain,
You answer inner promptings to create
Spell out in feathered movement far more sure
A pattern humans cannot imitate
Save when purest inspiration may dictate,
Though never with such ease or lack of pain.
Yet all living things obey the same iron law
And that which makes the eager blackbird make,
Makes everyone of us sometime in life
An artist bent on harmonising strife –
And from the crudest things about us raise
Some structure both of use and praise.

Omar Sabbagh

The Bird In The Tree

It was as if
a film
of surreal gloss
Circled the triangle
Of that figure – so black
It was purple;
a painter's wicked slash
Of coal-grey across
the black breast,
a heart-thick
diagonal,
The only sign of life, or of interest
In the same…

The bird in the tree
seemed lost,
Foundering, a perched dream through a crack
In the seam
of the workaday reality.
                    Was it silly of me to see

That weird
White-lined aura that freed
The bird from the custom of the picture?

As though some wraith, a slim cure,
Some rapier
Of sublime pencil
Had tracked its shape
To a strangely-mental
Completion –

it was no more bird,
no more simple
Avatar / epigone
of the reptile,

But a voice in black in the white world,
But a voice on the eye that the eye heard.

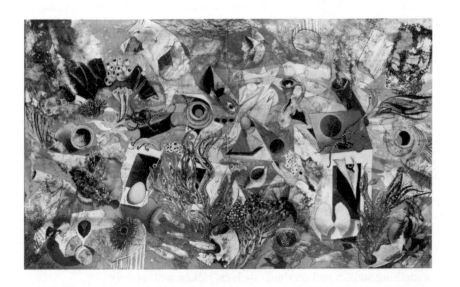

CHOSEN BROADSHEET POETS

Patrick Wright, 35. is a writer and academic living and working in Manchester. After his PhD on the sublime at the University of Manchester, he has taught English and Art History at the University of Manchester, University of Salford, MMU and the Open University. He currently teaches 'The Arts Past and Present' and 'Voices, Texts and Material Culture' with the OU: humanities modules, which include Creative Writing. Thus far, he is author of two books and several academic articles.

The Ghost Room

All day she's been at the craft table punching butterflies
out of stolen *Vogue* issues. She's making me a sconce
to say sorry – sorry for the abuse blamed on the moon –
one panel of flatpack upped with usual flair into
something stellar; and on those shelves, ricked with gravity –
'jenga' – she's arranged for us a mirror:

Her chandelier stuns like a jellyfish, wedding dress
gauze wrapped improv round the fitting. It sways a little.
Then the mannequin propped by her balcony, 'Ernest.'
We talk of him as if he's our son (since we understand
by now we aren't going to have one), and our daughter's
the Bratz doll who basks in a fairy castle.

Nowhere is anything sane – and this is us, the room
built on schisms. And beneath the frolics
I can't help wonder why her children don't make contact.
Yes, this is us, where handbags amass like surrogate wombs;
we're in a world of white-themed-things,
where the joke begins to wear itself thin.

Nullaby

The only sounds this evening are the solitary
pulse of an electric aromatic diffuser
and occasional sea-echo from the fridge.
The diffuser purrs in the hearth corner
I need to brighten by clearing out her
batik scarves – black-starred with mold –
driftwood planks for *doll prosthetics*
and a hundred keepsake carrier bags.
    The motor fans out a nimbus of steam
lit by a revolving door of gels – blues,
pinks, cerise. Her concoction still somehow
knocks me out. Christmas oil, lavender, tea tree.
    Higher towards the ceiling throbs
an infrared lamp – a binary companion? –
not some common-or-garden sixty watt thing
but a heat-emitting glowworm
she nursed my sacroiliac with. It casts the room
as a boudoir, a private red light district.

Outside the security bulb clicks on for a minute.
Squinting out the window
a refuse sack of shoes. Naked back to bed,
the pillow's indent, a single hair, a scattering
of hearts *punkt* out of what I called junk;
for her something to upcycle…
    And the down-cycling of us, trashing
our trust, finding the sinister in a snowflake –
a borderline state? an inner script?
Is she in London with the lunatics?
Is she in the care of the services?
Couldn't stand her gaslighting the flat.
    No arguing over *exclusive*. No texts firing
gatling gun. No love by a thousand cuts.
Headfucked till I switched her off. And still
the psychic stabs: *you have destroyed me…*
Her hour of need, I refused a key, let her
sleep on benches, walk out into traffic…

No clock ticks – an iPod charges
with the alarm set for eight on chimes.
Those grate the least. For now
the milk float roads are less lit than dreams –
dreams of finding her: an asylum visit
where no one speaks. I close my eyes,
come close to agreeing the gust really *is*
the ghost of a train, confuse words for things,
fear the slightest creak of wood contracting
when the boiler sleeps.
    A car slushes the latest downpour
and strobes its headlights down the wardrobe –
a friend for a second...
    And I'm at it again. How there's nothing
to find sane this red-eyed morning –
the upped dimmer-switch of dawn. How thoughts
find reflections in unwashed clothes on the carpet.
How the sun seems to rise without intent.

Elisions

Facing you in the loggia, as you hand-comb
your sputnik-shaped bed hair –
the tuft especially you say is my fault –
I guess this is intimacy. On the surface
husband and wife, minutiae and erogenous zones
all known, the familiar eyes I wake to,
half-moon and dopily assured, the morning
ritual of Earl Grey and powdered milk,
your query about the sun, sieved
through voile curtains, or some dark
surreal you dragged out of your dream.
    Is it for me to discern where the day-
light begins? Certain words go unsaid
in the dictionary, ones I've bracketed
as they remind us of the *other woman*,
of London, clonazepam; the episodes
we hope are behind us. Have I silenced
that part of you – of phantasms, threats,
fugues, of analysing words like *concubine*
over and over? Or does it stay remote?
    This is for your sake: not saying words like *fox*
(that's her surname), once chained to *Fuchs*,
then *fucks*, as you felt those words betrayed
my *philandering side*. And now no signs
as we breakfast before another act. To check
each word, not trigger you, reflect on it fast,
think at all times of your otherness – the -osis.
I was faithful all along.

Sarah Lindon's poems have appeared in *Magma, Poetry Wales, Scintilla, Seam, Stand* and *The Reader* and in *Tokens for the Foundlings* ed. Tony Curtis (Seren, 2012). In 2012 she completed an MPhil in writing at what was then the University of Glamorgan. She is 34 and lives and works in London.

I am a group of shadows

I alight from the dark and pass,
like a folded puppet, over the doorframe.
I fan and fall across the room,
indicate a set of disparate directions.

Now and then I peel off a self,
which prompts you to look
to see what you are seeing,
to search, perhaps, for a lit double.

I make you question
the location of lampposts,
the setting sun,
the physics of light,
the house's wiring,
if only for a flicker
of a moment.

When you tire of me,
as you soon do, I pull myself together
to a single figure
and withdraw to a shaded corner, or blur big
and seep across the ceiling,
or I turn on my profile and edge along
the wainscot's foot
and back outside.

I haven't yet found the body
I am to hang myself around.
In my sprawling spare time, solo
or dispersed, I watch actors
work out their blocking, or
I worry at the scenes of crimes.

Sunplay

sunlight places office workers
along the canal, spaced out a little,
like dolls on a designer's model

a man talking on the phone,
hand on hip, the woman
ankles crossed, book in lap

or perhaps I put them there,
in this arrangement
and when I look back and see

two placed too close together
I will reach down across the sun
and nudge one along

who will break into a run
but fail to sweat because the heat
I forgot to turn it on

and she will vanish
around the bend opposite the barge
and I will let her go

because I am also fleeing
the huge clumsy hands of my mind
passing over the world

and I turn back to something
humdrum, a spreadsheet say,
where I may think confined

Bat

The bat extends its hand of a wing
with which it grabs and throws the air
the way a conductor plays an orchestra,
it leans on and elbows and strokes each current,
barging and dancing its erratic acrobatics
through webs of ricocheting sonar.
Dog-faced screecher, little live nightmare,
it veers from pell-mell mastery of darkness
to its clotted hive of heads and hardened leather,
hung practically like so many umbrellas,
joints and jaws heavy with potential,
half-beast, half-insect, in eerie suspension.

Cricket

It finds its pitch and finds its pitch,
sets out its armature and lets its jitters keen,
distracted music, too-tentative Stravinsky,
percussively repeating, trying to scaffold
itself, a Pompidou riddled with arthritis,
proud-eyed but prone to shock, crouched
pre-palpitation until sprung, then travelling
with stickish flurry, landing an antique heartbeat.
Even in its pomp its sap is spare, poor threadbare
puppet. But do not pity it. This Giacometti
consumes the space around it, eats the very air
out of enormous appetite and terror.

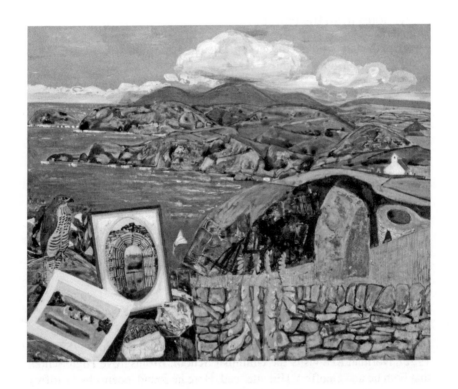

NOTES FOR BROADSHEET POETS

A few notes from the editor

> Trim the lamp; polish the lens; draw, one by one, rare
> coins to the light...
>
> Geoffrey Hill, *Mercian Hymns (XIII)*

What better advice to anyone who writes poetry, young or old?

'I write poetry' is different from the big claim 'I am a poet'. It has always seemed to me to be such an arrogance to refer to oneself as 'a poet'. So many people do just this without a blush, in particular those who have graduated from Creative Writing Schools. Geoffrey Hill surely agreed with Yves Bonnefoy who said, 'One should not call oneself a poet. It would be pretentious. It would mean that one has resolved the problems poetry presents. *Poet* is a word one can use when speaking of others, if one admires them sufficiently. If someone asks me what I do, I say I'm a critic, or a historian.'

The School boy Geoffrey Hill

In the Geoffrey Hill: Sixtieth Birthday issue of *Agenda* (Spring/Summer 1992), Norman Rea visits the Grammar School, Bromsgrove High School that both he and Geoffrey Hill attended. Here he found poems by Geoffrey in the school magazine. From Hill's earliest humorous juvenilia on boating, fishing and football, accomplished in rhyme and rhythm, to his more mature verse which possessed a 'new power', a leap in maturity, it became evident from the fifth form upwards, as evidenced in his poem 'Fotheringhay, 1587' published in the school magazine in 1949, that 'Geoffrey Hill was a major presence in our literary world and was developing as a very good poet indeed'. With apologies to Geoffrey, we re-print this 'poem' here as an inspiration (or perhaps a disincentive!) to all young 'poets' who will be able to tease out many hallmarks of Hill's later work.

Fotheringhay, 1587

i

The rain-flaked sky-wheel rubs the
Dove-tailed shingle off the stall,
The pied mare heaves and moans in foal.

The iron-keeper's scaffold holds the
Whirling circle of the wall.
Out of its orbit shoots the soul.

Circles start and stop in pain,
    But I –
Until the axe-arc fall again –
    Am whole.

ii

Morning moved the image nearer
To the constant queen, and clearer
Came the rays of life to sere her.

Praying gave the image grace,
But dread of death usurped its place:
Fear wiped its hand across her face

And passed; for dying on the bleak
Scaffold, she saw what all men seek.
But then it was too late to speak.

iii

The elder doffed its cap of mist. The wind
Drummed through the snaring branches of the wood
Till the black-laced birches bobbed on their toes
Like eager children at a festival.

And craning forward they saw the sun, mounting
With firm step to her expectant zenith, poise
At the turn of the stair and brazenly
Lean on a bannister of cloud, waiting...

Waiting until her desire died. Lust waned
With the wind, and the drooped birches dozed as
The moon crept like a little dog to lie
Between the head and shoulders of the earth.

Here already the teenage poet shows his skill in the use of 'negative capability', placing himself in the mind and body of the queen. Here too, with a concise narrative that changes in tone and mood, he approaches questions of mortality: 'she saw what all men seek.//But then it was too late to speak' and intimates his holistic view of the cosmos with the sun and moon which frame the death of the queen. Images are startlingly vivid and original, intensified by devices such as hitched-together words, personification of the trees, sun, similes and metaphors, all contributing to the overall music of the poem. The rhyming triplets in part ii seem ironic as it is here that the queen dies on the scaffold. Likewise in i where there is a subtle intricate patterning of rhyme with the second lines of the first two triplets rhyming, and also the third lines. The broken lines pre-empt her broken life, yet paradoxically resound in triumph since the queen remains 'whole'.

Omar Sabbagh, a former young *Agenda* Broadsheet poet, and now an established essayist and poet with several collections to his name, and a novel about to be published, looks closely here at Geoffrey Hill's poem, 'Genesis'.

As far as we know, human beings are unique in the animal kingdom, in so far as they write and are capable of writing poetry. And poetry, here, may stand in for all symbolic use of language, language which transcends the function of mere communication. How did we get this capacity? And, more significantly, why did we get this capacity? Even if we are merely the last in a slow gradating line of other animals, wherefore this gift? For surely there is something radically different, at-odds with the behaviours of other animals, in telling stories. And, in poetry, there is something expressed quite beyond the atomic breakdown of words or sounds or signs that indicate mere survival needs. When we read a great poem, it is surely more than its mechanical breakdown – because it means; it is more than the perfectly-parsed definitions of all its separate words. So: wherefore – or why – this prodigal capacity?

Perhaps it was God? Which is to say, a gift lit in us from within – dubbed tellingly in the Western tradition: a Word, a Logos, or a Ratio – from a transcendent Person or Mind? Whether this is the truth of the matter or not (and none will ever know), the idea of humanity being special, marked-out, in this sense, is of a piece with the religious notion of God's creation being *ex nihilo*; and this model is in my view the most apt pattern upon which to model our own, mortal, poetic creation. I'd like to discuss the first poem in Geoffrey Hill's first collection, *For The Unfallen*, titled, 'Genesis,' to elicit this view.

The declarative poetic voice, a man, is both before and after Man. There are five sections to the poem, representing within them six days of creation. The poet is thus one behind creation – *both in both senses*. The poet is also, presumably, writing from the perspective of the day of rest, one day beyond the content; *as well as* day by day, section by section.

The first word of the first line is 'Against' ('the burly air I strode') and the first word of the second line is 'Crying' ('the miracles of God.') Two double entendres then: or irony as well as gravitas. The poetic voice is set into relief by and sets into relief 'God'; and the miracles of creation are both cried/lauded by the voice and are of a nature to cry/weep.

Throughout the poem, the difference between a 'Logos' and what George Steiner in *Real Presences* calls 'the epi-logue' is adverted to; the difference between being an originating Person and being a latecomer or artifact of that very origin; the difference between a language that references a given world, already objectively 'out there,' and a language that creates reality as it's expressed. The poet is in a sense the 'God' of the poem and (set off) 'Against' Him.

And first I brought the sea to bear
Upon the dead weight of the land;
And waves flourished at my prayer,
The rivers spawned their sand.

These are the third to sixth lines of this first section. The sea is like the spirit breathed into the letter, the 'dead weight.' If the waves flourish at the poet's 'prayer' though, he clearly isn't the Creator but dependent on such. Similarly, just as spirit is breathed into dead letter, so, 'the river spawned its sand;' namely, the solid comes after the fluid. Again, a force-field in which Creator and creature are fudged, or made ambivalent. '[S]pawned' is both realistic, given the grainy nature of sand, and loaded with Satanic intents. In a similar manner, for all their visceral vitality and vibrancy as penned, 'the tough pig-headed salmon' towards the end of this first section, strive, 'To reach the steady hills above.' Which is to say realism and surrealism, gravitas and irony, creature and Creator beyond the bounds of the senses or the possible are one and many.

In the second section the poet stands and sees the violence of the 'osprey' 'with triggered claw' laying 'the living sinew bare' on the 'shore.' The poet is both witness of creation and penning that very act of witnessing. He is both first person and third person. Below, the 'hawk's' 'deliberate stoop' and its being 'Forever bent upon the kill,' is another description of visceral violence which is ratified by the assonance and consonance, the ruddiness and density of the language. But more than this, this animal violence is perhaps a metaphor for the torsion lived and evinced in poetic creativity, that plucking from the infinite dark both within oneself and within language. Creation is both *ex nihilo* – the poet's unique perspective in space and time, say – and work upon something that came before, and that comes after, namely, language. Self and Other imply each other, like life and death.

So when we read in the third section of the 'ashes of the sea' we are reminded of the hermeneutic interpenetration of life and death, or the two trees which might be signified by what the poet calls, 'the unwithering tree,' that of knowledge and that of life. Indeed the beginning of the next, fourth section, enacts this antinomy by talking of the rising 'phoenix' (a pre-Christian redemption in contrast to the later-invoked Christ) as 'burning' 'cold as frost.' This bird is 'lost' and 'pointless' we learn, so that on the 'fifth

146

day' the poet returns to more mundane reality 'To flesh and blood and the blood's pain.' This: just before the final section which introduces the more humane or inhumane redemption of Christ and the Christian tradition. But even here, there is paradox: 'the blood's pain.' What could this mean but, again, the pain of the flesh, *as well as* the pain of pain, a bit like the thought of thought, which is one definition of God, Logos; thus, here, again, the alternating of the poet as before and after God and himself.

In the fifth section the poetic voice 'rides' 'about the works of God,' and we are faced with another double entendre: the poet is all 'about' the works of God, lauding them, marvelling and also topographically going around them: he both names them and reflects upon them. And though men are made free by Christ's 'blood', and though no 'bloodless myth will hold' – both of which justify the content and the expression of the poet – despite this 'weight' we, that is, those discussed by the poet and the poet himself, by turns, are 'bones that cannot bear the light.' In other words we are epilogues to a thorough Logos. We don't follow in His footsteps, so walk in darkness I suppose. And yet, we *certainly have* followed the stepping feet of the poet.

When in the last section Hill writes, 'By blood we live, the hot, the cold, / To ravage and redeem the world...' he expresses again the paradox of eternity and temporal existence, life and death. Or, if you like, just as in the implicit contrast between the mythic 'phoenix' and 'Christ', the contrast between Manicheanism and the more properly Christian view. One suggests that matter pre-existed creation, the other suggests that creation was the work of something out of nothing. Similarly, the poet is as original as the language allows him to be.

In a way, this poem invokes the basic question of metaphysics, 'Why is there not nothing?' When we ask it in language, as a (mortal) sentence, we commit a pragmatic contradiction: just to put 'why' or indeed 'w' is already to assume some thing. We cannot practically get behind the positivity of our own existence; we are inexorably 'thrown' in(to) this world, to use Heidegger's phrase; and yet, if, just if there is the possibility of the meaningful thought *separate from* the material sentence (different in different languages after all), then meta-physics, or the reality of the world out there, is possible and salvaged. There is a spirit behind, through the letter.

If we just had physics, we'd be as clueless or story-less as the rest of the animal kingdom. If you like, the ability to question with a 'Why?', just as the ability to posit (though not access demonstrably) our own nothingness, sunders us from the rest of the material earth with as much of an absolute break as the very idea of creation out of nothing. For 'Why?' means an incipient story: the possibility of *poesis*: con-figuration; 'Why?' means the forthcoming constructions of the imagination; 'Why?' makes us symbolic, not merely literal beings. The rest of the animal kingdom doesn't tell stories, write poetry; as far as we know, they only communicate, functionally. And the paradox elicited so far is parsed here by the question: is this difference between us merely contingent, or is it essential? Are we the poetic creature par excellence, because we were made to be such, authors authored? Or, and at the same time, will we find out in five hundred or five thousand years an Odyssey spoken by the dolphins? This is the humane question posed and considered by Hill's poem, if implicitly.

And yet: can we 'bear' the light? Again, as throughout, the idea of 'weight' is paradoxically redolent: gravity in a physical sense throughout speaking to metaphysical gravity. At the last, unlike God, we are not able to wholly embody both: first person and third person perspectives at the same time – the given facts or data of the world, and their meanings for us. Our meaning-fuelled mortality means that we are essentially dissociated (thus, *pace* Eliot, essentially 'metaphysical'). It is our living in the rupture between the two – what is and what it means – that is the source of our drama and creativity.

God, on the other hand, and to put it in an iconic way, 'Is that He Is' – a tautology, with no dramatic or poetic tension; the 'tide's pull' (surreally) mentioned in the poem is how the poet as human animal needs must 'strive' towards (and is also emergent from, surely) silence.

Shanta Acharya reviews *Daodejing Laozi* – *A New Version in English by* Martyn Crucefix (Enitharmon Press, 2016)

A prize-winning translator and poet, Martyn Crucefix is a teacher of English who regularly publishes thought-provoking reviews and articles on his poetry blog. Having translated Rainer Maria Rilke's *Duino Elegies* and *Sonnets to Orpheus* with great success, this version of *Daodejing* extends his repertoire, illustrating his range and skill as a translator. Laozi, the author of *Daodejing*, is said to have despaired of the 'world's venality and corruption', but was persuaded to leave a record of his thoughts as a parting gift. The poems 'still vivid, astonishingly fresh, irresistible' were used as an aid to teaching from as far back as the 7th century BCE. However, the poems are not to be read as a handbook, nor as an instructional scripture, but as 'inspiration'. In his Introduction, Crucefix informs us these poems 'freely given at a point of change, a gateway to new experience' are 'an inspired outpouring of poetry as much as a moral and political handbook'.

In his version of *Daodejing*, Crucefix adheres to the traditional division between the 'Way' and the 'Power', enabling him 'to explore the nature of the Way before considering its more specific manifestations' in the Power. He also adopts a style that makes the original feel contemporary. The poems are 'unpunctuated, flowing, untrammelled' (Penelope Shuttle) enhancing their simple, authentic and paradoxical quality, drawing the reader into its message which is universally relevant. As Crucefix points out in his Introduction, 'we seem to hear Laozi writing a kind of poetry which enthusiastically accepts that its profound and heartfelt messages are inevitably compromised by the need to express them in the form of language, hence demanding that it employ a variety of technical manoeuvres, that it stays light on its feet'.

The unexpected opening sets the tone, reminding us not only of the limitations and imperfections of words/ language with which concept the book also ends ('Store' Chapter 81). It reminds us 'the Dao is not an individual entity, still less anything divine, it is more a mode of being that is all encompassing, a phenomenal, an existential primacy':

> – that the path I can put a name to
> cannot take me the whole way
>
> words I am capable of using
> are not the words that will remain

heaven and earth spring from wordlessness
what can be named is no more

than the nursery where ten thousand things
are raised each in their own way

The opening dash suggests both a continuation and an elision, and the relative pronoun, 'that', draws our attention to the path that one cannot put a name to, nor can it take us 'the whole way'. We learn that 'heaven and earth spring from wordlessness'. These lines from 'Nursery', Chapter 1, go on to say the Dao gives rise to 'ten thousand things', each raised in their own way, suggesting the Dao is the 'mother of all things'. ('Of all things', Chapter 25). The Dao is a vessel to be drawn from, the bottomless source of all things ('Something greater', Chapter 4). It is also the uncarved block of wood that has inherent within it all things that have been, are, will be ('Uncarved Wood', Chapter 15). It is 'the flood-gate from which flows greater truth' ('Nursery', Chapter 1).

The poems can be seen from multiple – 'epistemological, temporal, perceptual, political or environmental' – perspectives, though none of these exhaust its real nature. 'It is not subject to time yet contains it. It is never fixed. It is ever-here, both omnipresent and unchanging. We might be tempted to say the Dao is the substratum of all things,' says Crucefix. It reminds us of the great Unknown which is the essence of all being. The Dao is beyond conception and so beyond any conventional use of language, the limits of which constitute a recurring motif.

The Dao manifests several female qualities; the teacher reflects this in her quietness, passivity, sensitivity, lack of overt force ('Raw material, Chapter 27). By representing the teacher as wholly feminine – as 'personification of the Dao itself and as its incarnation in actual human form, a mother figure, a female teacher, a friend – Crucefix stamps his individuality in interpreting the original text. When the true teacher emerges, no matter how detached, unimpressive, even muddled she may appear, Laozi assures us 'there are treasures beneath'.

The primary concern of the text is how our growing awareness of the Dao shapes our personal lives. In the 'Three treasures' (Chapter 67) we are urged 'to be compassionate frugal to lack ambition'. As 'only those who feel compassion are truly brave/ only the frugal know sincere generosity/ only one reluctant to grasp power/ is properly capable of government'. In each of these manifestations of human behaviour, the ego is diminished if not relinquished, and there is a corresponding rise in one's awareness of others and the world, a kind of wise passivity. We are to act 'Like water'

(Chapter 8), flowing passively, dispassionately towards lower ground in both personal and political spheres ('Influence', Chapter 66).

Crucefix's versions reveal 'an astonishing empathy with what they have to say about good and evil, war and peace, government, language, poetry and the pedagogic process' (Introduction). Laozi suggests the teacher's role is to 'show, facilitate, enthuse, give space, watch and approve'. We must be honest, be ourselves, give the tools, give opportunities, do our job well, but then let go, don't dwell. Our role is to sympathise and connect, shed light, provide 'indirect direction'. And the best teacher's ambition, as spelt out in 'Store' (Chapter 81), is 'to sharpen not sever/ via the deed undone/ without rules to govern.' In 'Dazed' (Chapter 49), we learn:

the true teacher is like a poet
who has no self to speak of
using the self of others as his own

This idea of selflessness is found in various systems of thought – from Hinduism to Sufism. We are also reminded of Keats' notion of Negative Capability, 'when a man is capable of being in uncertainties, mysteries, doubts, without any irritable reaching after fact and reason'. In his letter of 27 October 1818 to Richard Woodhouse, Keats wrote: 'As to the poetical character itself…it is not itself–it has no self–it is everything and nothing'… This aspect of being a poet/teacher is what it means to be human, to serve others while growing in mindfulness. In 'Doing Nothing' (Chapter 47), we learn: 'ever mindful/ in doing nothing/ she pursues/ her goals'. A book for all times, the ideal society we could live in is described in 'The Commonwealth' (Chapter 80). The poem ends with: 'the people of my country/ would grow wise/ they would age without knowing/ the restless desire to visit', the treasures of compassion, frugality and lack of ambition being rare gifts for us who live in interesting times.

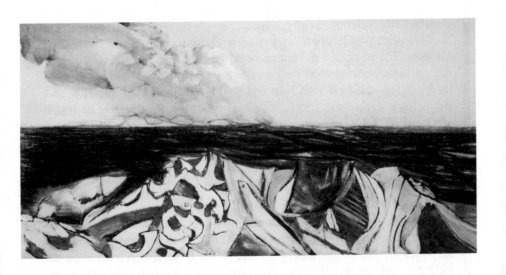

Yves Bonnefoy: June 24th, 1923 – July 1st, 2016

In one sweep of the scythe, the grim reaper gathered in two great poets, Geoffrey Hill, celebrated and commemorated in this issue of *Agenda*, and in his 93rd year, Yves Bonnefoy, who died a few hours after, on the morning of 1st July. The two poets did not know each other, and everything separates their practice, except total devotion to the craft, and a tenacious faith in its efficacy – the hard-won 'sad and angry consolation' of late Hill, and Bonnefoy's early 'manifesto', in a famous essay of 1959, where he states, '*Je voudrais réunir, je voudrais identifier presque la poésie et l'espoir*'. Both poets also drew deep on resources found in childhood – Hill obliquely in *Mercian Hymns* and more explicitly in *The Triumph of Love* and the 'Parentalia' poems, Bonnefoy explicitly in criticism, but also in the two great texts of self-analysis, *L'Arrière-pays* (1972) and his final prose work, completed only months before his death, *L'Écharpe rouge*. The latter is an astounding, and disturbing exegesis, in the smallest detail, of every line of a fragmentary, but obscure poem, 'given' to him as early as 1964, and it centres around the disturbing 'silence of the father', who worked on the railways, and was increasingly estranged from his bookish and brilliant son.

In a lapidary, oft-quoted formulation, Bonnefoy said that 'the task of the poet is to show us a tree, before the intellect tells us that it is one', and again, he once likened the apprehension of *présence*, a frequent term in his work, as akin to getting lost in a forest, when the trees, and their density, can take on an altogether more fearful, and hence less 'conceptual' aspect. A certain tree he fixes, during the burial service of a grandparent in the Lot, or the vision of a peasant stooped at work, framed in a window passed one night – these things seem to have sunk deeply into the poet's young psyche. They will often recur in different, sometimes mythological, guises, apprehended '*dans l'absolu*' ; but crucially, and after struggle, these presences become friendly, affirmative, and joined into an organic whole – the reverse that is of Mallarmé's 'flower' which, no sooner enounced, floats free of all specificity. A paradox in Bonnefoy (there are many) is his insistence on specificity while employing in his poetry a 'purified' vocabulary in which certain words – fire, dream, light, a barque on the dark river, stone – accrue weight. A glance at Hill's work, with its vast, recherché vocabulary, and armoury of allusion, could not give more credence to another of the French poet's famous distinctions – that the English language operated like an all-reflecting Aristotelian mirror, and French like a crystal sphere – distilling and refining.

Bonnefoy, a devoted student of English, in many ways his desired 'other' language for the reasons given above, translated Keats and Yeats, and ten Shakespeare plays, complete with long, idiosyncratic commentary, notably on the rôle and sacrifice of Shakespeare's women ; in this alone he commands our respect – he belongs in the great tradition of French Shakespeareans – Victor Hugo & son, Stendhal, Baudelaire among them. In the 'sixties he taught at several distinguished American universities, and met and married an American artist, Lucy Vines. It was also with her that he discovered his 'true place' (*vrai lieu*) – another crucial and persistent element in the work – Valsaintes, a deserted abbey in Provence in which they camped out and tried to restore, at least partially, through several enchanted summers that Bonnefoy celebrates in his two major affirmative collections *Pierre écrite* (1965) and *Dans le leurre du seuil* (1975). In these, Bonnefoy emerges as a great poet of the earth, and they also contain rapturous love poetry. In the end the couple had to abandon the house to the 'nettles and the stones', but that apparently prolonged experience of presence seems to have emboldened Bonnefoy in his increasingly sanguine poetics of hope. It might be said that – and in this the contrast is so sharp with Geoffrey Hill – the struggle goes out of the poems themselves (until the last books, which contain material of a much more personal nature) – as they state their epiphanies. For me, the great books of struggle are the early ones, especially *Hier régnant désert* (1953 – beautifully translated into English by Tony Rudolf) and the prose meditation *L'Arrière-pays* (1972), my own translation of which appeared in 2012. But the critic in Bonnefoy was always wary, sceptical, and never sought or believed in transcendental revelation. As he said in his inaugural *leçon* on his accession to the Chair of Poetics at the Collège de France in 1981 (the successor to Paul Valéry and Roland Barthes) – 'there can be no being, unless we wish there to be being' and that it is the 'relation to the other that is at the origin of being'.

Yves Bonnefoy's own death, his 'assent to mortality' – from the start, a foundational tenet of his poetics – can only be described as a *leçon* to others, of the most humbling kind. It was almost papal: abandoning in extremis a final essay on his beloved Poussin, messages of *adieu* were then sent out, by the intermediary of his daughter Mathilde, individually to friends and collaborators, painters and publishers, including to his host of translators ; there were several moving final meetings at the hospice, details of the forthcoming *Pléiade* to be discussed, for Bonnefoy was always lucid about his work. And at the funeral, at Père Lachaise in Paris on 11 July, he addressed the assembled friends for the last time, in a long pre-recorded recitation of his last, testamentary poem, fittingly entitled 'Ensemble encore', together still.

Stephen Romer

BIOGRAPHIES

An internationally published poet, critic, reviewer and scholar, **Shanta Acharya** is the author of ten books. Her *New and Selected Poems* is to be published by HarperCollins (India) in January 2017. Educated at Oxford and Harvard, her work has been featured in major publications, including *Poetry Review*, *PN Review*, *The Spectator*, *The Guardian Poem of the Week*, *Edinburgh Review*, *The Bloodaxe Book of Contemporary Indian Poets*, *Journal of Postcolonial Writing*, *Asia Literary Review*, *The Little Magazine*, *The HarperCollins Book of English Poetry*, *Language for a New Century: Contemporary Poetry from the Middle East, Asia & Beyond*. In 1996, she founded 'Poetry in the House', and has been responsible for hosting monthly readings at Lauderdale House, in London. She has twice served on the board of trustees of The Poetry Society, UK. www.shantaacharya.com

Timothy Adès, rhyming translator-poet, has books of Jean Cassou and Robert Desnos, from *Agenda* and also from Arc Publications; and Victor Hugo from Hearing Eye and Arvelo from Shearsman. Alfonso Reyes, Brecht, and Sikelianós are other favourites. He has written lipograms, notably Shakespeare's Sonnets without the letter e.

Louis Aragon 1897-1982, major French poet, novelist, translator and cultural commentator, decorated in both wars, author of over a hundred books, wrote this poem in 1945 when the ashes of Robert Desnos were brought from Terezin. Both had been in the Surrealist group round André Breton, and were active in the Resistance.

David Attwooll's first full collection, *The Sound Ladder,* was published in April 2015 by Two Rivers Press. His work has appeared in several magazines and anthologies, and he was one of the winners of the 2013 Poetry Business pamphlet prize with *Surfacing* (smith/doorstop). *Ground Work* (Black Poplar, 2014) followed, a pamphlet illustrated by Andrew Walton. David works in publishing and drums in a street band.

Elizabeth Barton read English at Christ's College, Cambridge, after which she moved countries and had a family. She has worked as an English teacher and has written freelance articles published in *The Times* and *The Catholic Herald*. She lives in Surrey and is a member of Mole Valley Poets.

William Bedford is a prize-winning poet and novelist. Red Squirrel Press published his *The Fen Dancing* in 2014. His poem 'The Journey' won First Prize in the 2014 *London Magazine* International Poetry Competition. Another poem 'Then' won First Prize in the 2014 Roundel Poetry Competition. In the autumn of 2015, Red Squirrel Press published *The Bread Horse*, a new collection of poems.

Sharon Black is originally from Glasgow but now lives in the Cévennes mountains of southern France where she organizes writing retreats. She has been published widely and was runner-up in the Troubadour Poetry Prize in 2013. Her first collection, *To Know Bedrock,* was published by Pindrop Press in 2011. Her second, *The Art of Egg*, was out with Two Ravens Press in 2015. www.sharonblack.co.uk

Nick Burbridge is an Anglo-Irish poet, playwright, novelist, journalist, short story and song writer, who lives in Brighton. He is the author of three books of poetry: *On Call* (Envoi Poets, 1994), *All Kinds Of Disorder* (Waterloo, 2006) and *The Unicycle Set,* (Waterloo, 2011). His plays include *Dirty Tricks* (Soho Theatre), *Vermin* (Finborough), and *Cock Robin* (Verity Bargate Award Runner-up), and have been broadcast on BBC Radio. He is an award-winning songwriter.

Vuyelwa Carlin was born in South Africa, brought up in Uganda, came to England to read English at Bristol and has lived in Shropshire for many years. She has published four collections to date; the fifth, *Long Shadows,* published by Poetry Salzburg, will be out shortly. She has had poems published in many magazines and anthologies.

Peter Carpenter is the co-director of Worple Press and a teacher at Tonbridge School; he has had seven collections of poems published, most recently *Peace Camp* (Maquette, 2015) and *Just Like That* (Smith/Doorstop, 2012).

Martin Caseley is a teacher, poet and essayist. He lives in Lincolnshire and essays have appeared in *PN Review* and *Agenda*. Some recent poems have appeared in *'Yesterday's Music Today'*, published by the Knives Forks and Spoons Press.

David Cooke won a Gregory Award in 1977. *A Murmuration*, his fourth collection was published by Two Rivers Press in 2015. His work has appeared in many journals in the UK, Ireland and beyond in *Agenda*, *Ambit*, *The Cortland Review*, *The Interpreter's House*, *The Irish Press*, *The London Magazine*, *Magma*, *The Manhattan Review*, *The Morning Star*, *New Walk*, *The North*, *Poetry Ireland Review*, *Poetry Salzburg Review*, *The Reader*, *The SHOp* and *Stand*. His next collection, *After Hours*, will be published by Cultured Llama in 2018. He is a co-editor of *The High Window*.

Peter Dale's most recent books of poems are *Local Habitation*, and *Diffractions: New and Selected Poems*, both published by Anvil Press, now part of Carcanet Press. He has also jointly written a book on dowsing with John Bowers, *Grounded*, Minilith Press, 2014, who also publish his current book of verse, *Aquatints*, obtainable from 11 Heol Y Gors, Whitchurch, Cardiff, CF14 1HF. He is now trying to finish what may well be his last book of verse.

Keith Grant (born 1930) is one Britain's greatest living landscape painters. He has travelled extensively, and has confronted the elements in order to produce extraordinary, resonant images of nature, especially in the north. Recently, he has preferred to recollect his experiences in the tranquillity of his studio in Norway, and works imaginatively to produce exciting series of what he considers to be 'autobiographical' paintings. He is represented by the Chris Beetles Gallery, St James's, London, which has held two highly successful solo shows of his work: 'Elements of the Earth' (2010) and 'Metamorphosis' (2016).

Graham Hardie is 43, lives near Glasgow and works as a gardener. His poetry has been published in *Agenda, Shearsman, The Interpreter's House, Gutter, The New Writer, Markings, Nomad, Cutting Teeth, The David Jones Journal, Cake* and online at *nth position* and *Ditch*.

David Harsent has published eleven volumes of poetry. *Legion* won the Forward Prize for best collection 2005; *Night* (2011) was triple short-listed in the UK and won the Griffin International Poetry Prize. His most recent collection, *Fire Songs*, won the 2014 T.S. Eliot Prize. Harsent has collaborated with a number of composers, though most often with Harrison Birtwistle, on pieces that have been performed at venues including the Royal Opera House, BBC Proms, the Aldeburgh Festival, The Concertgebouw, The London South Bank Centre, The Salzburg Festival, The Holland Festival and Carnegie Hall. Harsent is a Fellow of the Royal Society of Literature.

Jeremy Hooker's two most recent books are: *Scattered Light* (Enitharmon) and *Openings: A European Journal* (Shearsman). Shearsman will shortly publish his *Diary of a Stroke* and *Ancestral Lines* (a sequence of poems). As well as poetry and journals, he has published extensively on modern British and American poetry and Welsh writing in English.

Rosalind Hudis is a poet living in West Wales. Her publications include *Terra Ignota* (Rack press 2013) and *Tilt* (Cinnamon Press 2014) In 2015 she was highly commended in the Forward Prize for Poetry, was a runner-up in the Aesthetica Creative Writing Competition, and was placed first in the Cinnamon Press Single Poem Prize. She is an editor on *The Lampeter Review*.

W. D. Jackson's *Then and Now – Words in the Dark* (2002) and *From Now to Then* (2005) are published by Menard Press. *Boccaccio in Florence* (Shearsman, 2009) and *Afterwords* (Shoestring, 2014) are full-length selections from his work-in-progress, *Opus 3*. The pamphlet, *A Giotto Triptych*, was also published by Shoestring in 2014.

Dylan Jones has published two collections of poetry; *Dreaming Nightly of Dragons* (University of Salzburg 1996) and *Balances & Turns* (Umbrella Head 2011).

He has developed an interest in presenting his poetry visually as framed prints, and in October/November 2014 an exhibition of archival poem-prints *A Bird Flew By* was held in the Café Gallery, Aberystwyth Arts Centre. He sings and is a co-songwriter with mid-Wales romantic melancholics 'The Sheiling'.

Angela Kirby grew up in rural Lancashire, 1932, but now lives in London. The author of five books on cooking, gardening and related subjects, her poems are widely published and broadcast. In 1996 and 2001 she was the B.B.C.'s Wildlife Poet of the Year. Shoestring Press published her four collections: *Mr. Irresistible*, 2005, *Dirty Work*, 2008, *A Scent of Winter*, 2013, *The Days After Always, New and Selected Poems*, 2015. Much of her work has been translated into Romanian.

Gill Learner lives in Reading. Her poetry has won several awards and been widely published in journals, and in anthologies such as *Her Wings of Glass* and *Fanfare* (Second Light Publications, 2014 & 2015) and *The Day Destroyed* (Wilfred Owen Association, 2015). Her first collection, *The Agister's Experiment* (Two Rivers Press, 2011) was generously reviewed and her second, *Chill Factor* (June 2016) contains poems from *Agenda 48/3–4 & 49/1*.

John Robert Lee is a St. Lucian writer. His short stories and poems can be found in many journals and international anthologies. These include *Facing the sea* (1986), *The Penguin Book of Caribbean Verse* (1986), *The Faber Book of Contemporary Caribbean Short Stories* (1990), *The Heinemann Book of Caribbean Poetry* (1992), and *The Oxford Book of Caribbean Verse* (2005). Journals include *Bim; Callaloo; EnterText (UK); The New Voices (Trinidad & Tobago); Poetry Wales; Savacou; Small Axe; Trinidad & Tobago Review; Wasafiri (UK);), Review 81; World Poetry Portfolio #58 – Molossus, ArtsEtc (Barbados), Agenda, The Missing Slate, Prairie Schooner*. His poetry collections include: *Saint Lucian*

(1988), *Clearing ground* (1991), *Canticles* (2007), *Elemental* (2008), *Sighting* (2013), *City Remembrances* (2016). He has compiled a *Bibliography of Saint Lucian Creative Writing* 1948-2013 (2013), edited an anthology of St. Lucian poetry and art, *Roseau Valley and other poems* (2003) and co-edited *Sent Lisi: Poems and Art of Saint Lucia* (2014).

Christopher Meredith is a novelist and poet. He has been a steelworker and a schoolteacher and is an emeritus professor at The University of South Wales. His novel *Shifts* was shortlisted in 2014 for the title of Greatest Welsh Novel of All Time. His most recent novel is *The Book of Idiots*, and most recent collection is *Air Histories* (Seren).

Peter McDonald is the author of *Collected Poems* (2012), *Herne the Hunter* (2016) and *The Homeric Hymns* (2016).

Gill McEvoy's latest publications in print are *Rise*, Cinnamon press, 2013; *The First Telling*, Happenstance Press, 2014, which won the 2015 Michael Marks award. Gill runs regular and occasional poetry events in Chester. She is a Hawthornden Fellow.

Andrew McNeillie's most recent collection of poems is *Winter Moorings* (2014). He runs the Clutag Press, notably associated with Geoffrey Hill, and the magazine *Archipelago*.

W S Milne is an Aberdonian living in Surrey. His study on the early poetry of Geoffrey Hill was published in 1998. He has reviewed a number of Geoffrey Hill's collections of poetry for *Agenda*, and contributed essays in the special issues dedicated to his work.

John Mole lives in Hertfordshire and for many years ran The Mandeville Press with Peter Scupham. Recipient of the Gregory and Cholmondeley Awards, and the Signal Award for his poetry for children, his most recent publications are *The Point of Loss* (Enitharmon), and an online English/Romanian selection, *The Chemotherapy Experience* from Bucharest University's Contemporary Literature Press. He is also a jazz clarinettist, and has written the libretto for a community opera, *Alban*, first performed in St. Albans cathedral in 2009.

Tim Murdoch lives in the Alpujarras in Southern Spain. He devises yoga routines for people with back and other ailments. His poems have been in various magazines, most recently *Agenda* and the *London Magazine*; forthcoming in *PN Review*.

Paul Murray was born in Dublin in 1954. He now lives in Bray, Co. Wicklow. He has previously had poems published in *Agenda* and in the *Poetry Ireland Review*. He has also written school text books in the Irish language.

William Oxley was born in Manchester. His poems have been published in magazines and journals as diverse as *The New York Times, The Observer, The Spectator, The Independent, Agenda, Acumen, The London Magazine* and *Poetry Ireland Review*. A study of his poetry, *The Romantic Imagination*, appeared in 2005 from Poetry Salzburg. His *Collected and New Poems* came from Rockingham Press in 2014, and *Walking Sequence & Other Poems* from Indigo Dreams Publishing in 2015.

Jeremy Page has edited *The Frogmore Papers* since 1983. His short stories have been widely published, and he is the author of several collections of poems, most recently *Closing Time* (Pindrop, 2014). His translations of the Lesbia poems of Catullus were published as *The Cost of All Desire* by the Ashley Press in 2011. Jeremy Page lives in Lewes and works in the Centre for Language Studies at the University of Sussex.

David Pollard has been furniture salesman, accountant, TEFL teacher and university lecturer. He got his three degrees from the University of Sussex and has since taught at the universities of Sussex, Essex and the Hebrew University of Jerusalem where he was a Lady Davis Scholar. His doctoral thesis was published as: *The Poetry of Keats: Language and Experience* (Harvester and Barnes & Noble). He has also published *A KWIC Concordance to the Harvard Edition of Keats' Letters*, a novel, *Nietzsche's Footfalls* and five volumes of poetry, *patricides, Risk of Skin and Self-Portraits* (all from Waterloo Press), *bedbound* (from Perdika Press) and *Finis-terre* (from Agenda Editions). He has translated from Gallego, French and German. He has also been published in other volumes and in learned journals and poetry magazines. He divides his time between Brighton on the South coast of England and a village on the Rias of Galicia.

Angela Readman's collection *Strip* was published by Salt. More recently, her poems have won The Mslexia Poetry Competition, The Essex Poetry Prize, and The Charles Causey Prize. She also writes stories and won The Costa Short Story Award. Her debut story collection, *Don't Try This at Home* won a Saboteur Award in 2015.

Robert Richardson is a visual artist and writer. He is represented in *Artists' Postcards: A Compendium* (Reaktion Books, London), and in the past year has exhibited work in the Netherlands, Austria and Germany, as well as Britain. He is co-editor, with William Pratt, of *Homage to Imagism* (AMS Press, New York), and recently launched Poem *Flyer*, an innovative publishing project.

In 2014 **Tony Roberts** published his fourth collection of poems, *Drawndark*, and edited *Poetry in the Blood*. His essays, *The Taste in My Mind* , appeared in 2015, also from Shoestring Press.

Peter Robinson's novel *September in the Rain* is published by Holland House Books. His *Collected Poems* will appear from Shearsman Books in February 2017. He is currently completing a critical study called *The Sound Sense of Poetry* and a psycho-geographical homage to Robinson Crusoe entitled *The Constitutionals*. He is Professor of English and American Literature at the University of Reading and poetry editor for Two Rivers Press.

Stephen Romer is currently Fowler-Hamilton Visiting Research Fellow at Christ Church, Oxford. His translation of Yves Bonnefoy's *The Arrière-pays* was published by Seagull in 2012, and his anthology *French Decadent Tales* in 2013 (OUP World Classics).

Carol Rumens has published a number of collections of poetry, including. most recently, *De Chirico's Threads* (Seren, 2010) and *Animal People,* (Seren). Her awards include the Alice Hunt Bartlett Prize (with Thomas McCarthy), the Prudence Farmer Prize, and a Cholmondeley Award. She writes a regular poetry blog for Guardian Books Online, 'Poem of the Week', and teaches creative writing at Bangor University. She is a Fellow of the Royal Society of Literature.

Anne Ryland's first collection, *Autumnologist*, was shortlisted for The Forward Prize for Best First Collection in 2006, and her second collection, *The Unmothering Class*, was selected for New Writing North's Read Regional Campaign 2012. New poems have appeared in *Poetry Review*, *The North* and *Long Poem Magazine*, and earlier this year she won second prize in the Hippocrates Prize for Poetry and Medicine (Open Category).

Omar Sabbagh is a widely published poet and critic. His poetry and prose (critical and creative) have appeared in such venues as: *Poetry Review, PN Review, Poetry Ireland Review, The Reader, The Warwick Review, POEM, Kenyon Review Online, Poetry Wales, Stand, Wasafiri, The Wolf, Banipal, The London Magazine, The Moth, Lighthouse, Rusted Radishes, Envoi, New Welsh Review, Life Writing,* and elsewhere. His poetry collections include: *My Only Ever Oedipal Complaint* and *The Square Root of Beirut* (Cinnamon Press, 2010/12). A fourth collection, *To The Middle Of Love*, is forthcoming with Cinnamon Press in late 2016. His novel(la) set in and about Beirut, *Via Negativa: A Parable of Exile*, was published by Liquorice Fish Books in March 2016. A Dubai sequel to the latter, *From Bourbon to Scotch*, is set to be published in December 2016. Currently, he teaches at the American University in Dubai (AUD).

Will Stone is a poet, essayist and literary translator. His first poetry collection *Glaciation* (Salt, 2007), won the international Glen Dimplex Award for poetry in 2008. The sequel *Drawing in Ash*, was published in May 2011 (Salt) and Shearsman Books recently reissued these collections in new editions and published a third collection *The Sleepwalkers* in April 2016. His literary translations include works by Verhaeren, Rodenbach, Nerval, Trakl and Roth. Pushkin Press published his first English translation of Zweig's *Montaigne* in August 2015 and Zweig's *Messages from a lost world* in January 2016. He is currently writing a book on overlooked aspects of the cultural and historic landscape of Belgium.

Seán Street has published nine full poetry collections, the most recent being *Camera Obscura* (Rockingham Press, 2016). Prose includes *The Dymock Poets* (Seren 1994/14), *The Poetry of Radio: The Colour of Sound* (Routledge, 2013/14) and *The Memory of Sound: Preserving the Sonic Past* (Routledge, 2015/16). *Sound Poetics – Interaction and Personal Identity*, is forthcoming from Palgrave in 2017. His film-poem, *Elias*, was produced in 2015 by Red Balloon Productions. He is Emeritus Professor at Bournemouth University.

Jill Townsend lives in NE Hampshire. She has recently had work included in the anthology *Fanfare* from Second Light Publications and in the OUP book for parents and children *I Can Read!* Oxford Poetry for seven year olds.

Clive Wilmer has published six volumes of poetry with Carcanet Press, including *New and Collected Poems* (2012), and four volumes with Worple Press, including *Urban Pastorals* (2014). He is an Emeritus Fellow of Sidney Sussex College, Cambridge, and the Master of John Ruskin's Guild of St George. His essay on Geoffrey Hill, 'An Art of Recovery', appeared in *Agenda* in 1992.

Tony Conran:

Three Symphonies

(Agenda Editions 2016)

Tony Conran (1931-2013),
revered Welsh poet, was
a daring Modernist, in the
line of Pound, Bunting,
MacDiarmid and David Jones.

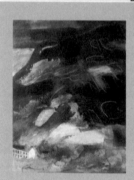

Three Symphonies

Tony Conran

   In his final group of
symphonies he explores life,
love, theology, creation,
creativity and even historical
themes using a wide range
of poetic and imaginative
techniques. The three
symphonies complement
and contrast with each other
and show the poet still at
the height of his imaginative power. The imagery
draws on science, religion, family life (in The Magi),
work (in Fabrics), the poetic and creative experience
(in Everworlds); displaying humour, wonder and
compassion for the human predicament.

   In his perceptive introduction to the poetry Jeremy
Hooker writes: '*Three Symphonies* draws on their
maker's life-story, but as part of the story of life itself,
and with an objectivity that subsumes personal emotion
in a larger rendering of human experience in relation to
the natural and divine creation. What Conran enacts in
these poems is a sacred drama.'

ISBN: 978-1-908527-25-7 Price £10